Understanding Advanced Statistics

D0965039

For Churchill Livingstone

Commissioning Editor: Alex Mathieson
Project Managers: Valerie Burgess and Ewan Halley
Senior Project Editor: Dinah Thom
Design Direction: Judith Wright
Sales Promotion Executive: Hilary Brown

Understanding Advanced Statistics

A Guide for Nurses and Health Care Researchers

Denis Anthony BA(Hons) MSc PhD RGN RMN RN(Canada) AMIEE
Lecturer, School of Health Sciences, The University of Birmingham, UK

Foreword by

Carolyn Hicks BA MA PhD PGCE CPsychol
Senior Lecturer in Psychology, School of Continuing Studies,
The University of Birmingham, UK

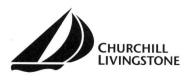

CHURCHILL
LIVINGSTONE

EDINBURGH LONDON NEW YORK PHILADELPHIA SYDNEY TORONTO 1999

CHURCHILL LIVINGSTONE
An imprint of Harcourt Brace and Company Limited

© Harcourt Brace and Company Limited 1999

 is a registered trademark of Harcourt Brace and Company Limited

First published 1999

ISBN 0 443 05933 0

British Library of Cataloguing in Publication Data
A catalogue record for this book is available from the British Library.

Library of Congress Cataloging in Publication Data
A catalogue record for this book is available from the Library of Congress.

Medical knowledge is constantly changing. As new information becomes available, changes in treatment, procedures, equipment and the use of drugs become necessary. The author and the publishers have, as far as it is possible, taken care to ensure that the information given in this text is accurate and up to date. However, readers are strongly advised to confirm that the information, especially with regard to drug usage, complies with current legislation and standards of practice.

The
publisher's
policy is to use
**paper manufactured
from sustainable forests**

Printed in China
EPC/01

Contents

Foreword

Health care provision internationally is currently undergoing radical change at all levels. Of particular relevance to this text are two major reforms – the increasing professionalization of the occupations allied to medicine and the shift towards an evidence rather than supposition-based health care culture. With respect to the first of these, the pressure to enhance the professional status of non-medical practitioners, such as nurses, physiotherapists, occupational and speech therapists, etc., has necessitated major changes to pre-registration training. The old apprenticeship models have been replaced by academically accredited courses that have a significant component of occupation-specific theory and research. Given that previous training was vocationally and practically oriented, the new curricula consequently created an immediate demand for high quality research that had the capacity to inform basic education and subsequent clinical practice. Moreover, as successive cohorts of graduates qualified under the new system, so the need for higher degrees and advanced post-basic education emerged. Together, these initiatives created an urgent requirement for both basic and more complex research output and research competence, neither of which had been considered essential under the previous training regime.

The second major issue of relevance to the present text is the global problem of how best to meet increasing demands for high quality health care within a context of diminishing funding. This, together with advances in technology, evolving policy initiatives, increasing professional accountability and litigation, means that there is no longer any room for clinical procedures that cannot be justified on cost and health effectiveness grounds. As a result, the concept of evidence-based practice has gathered momentum over the last decade as one means of encouraging the systematic delivery of clinical care that is properly grounded in scientifically derived research evidence.

Because clinical practice has traditionally been intuitive and ritualistic, the new evidence-based care culture represents a fundamental challenge to health professionals in every sector. Practitioners must now constantly reflect upon their care interventions in order to ensure that they can be vindicated by available research findings. Yet to integrate research with practice means that health professionals must have a sound knowledge of research methodologies. For those who qualified before the advent of the new research-oriented educational curricula as well as for more recent graduates, this fiat requires a commitment to engage with research as a routine part of their health care delivery. Research has become a byword for quality assurance.

Inevitably, both these reforms have meant that health carers must acquire and apply research skills as a customary part of their work. Cognizant of this, many texts offer a basic introduction to a range of research methodologies, designed to equip the professions with the essential competencies. Yet many of these books fail to meet the learning needs of the reader, either because the level is inappropriate or because the theory is not made properly relevant to the target audience. Moreover, with the increasing hold that research has established in health care delivery, there is now a need for a more advanced text that takes health care research beyond the fundamentals and into the more complex designs and data processing that are required both to enhance the quality of care provision, and to consolidate the complementary professional role of non-medical health carers. This book fulfils these aims.

Intending to develop to a more advanced yet pertinent level the research and statistical skills of the professions allied to medicine, Denis Anthony has produced a text that is relevant, accessible and encouraging. Statistics and research hold great fear for many people, but this structured approach to the topic offers a demystifying and confirming route through the more complex designs and the statistical and computing procedures required to analyse them. A considerable amount of health care research has moved beyond the type of data analysis that can comfortably be computed longhand or by calculators, requiring instead the flexibility, immediacy and complexity of statistical software packages. Yet many of us who completed our education before the advent of the IT revolution experience unmitigated fear when confronted with computers. Unfortunately, the vast majority of the available introductory books on computing that are intended to allay such fears, either assume an unrealistically high level of basic knowledge or alternatively have little apparent application to the reader's research or professional interests. Denis Anthony's book is clearly founded on long experience of teaching technophobes. By guiding the reader through sets of *occupationally relevant* instructions, illustrations and data sets, the reader can gain the expertise and the confidence to tackle both the more complex research designs that are pertinent to a wide range of health issues, as well as data inputting and computer analyses. Interspersed with these topics is guidance regarding their *application* and *interpretation* to field research, so that the researcher unfamiliar with a particular methodology can gain almost instant experience and insight. I have already used the draft to complete the computer analysis of two sets of data that hitherto I would have calculated by hand over a matter of weeks, sent out to a freelance statistician or abandoned altogether. The sense of mastery is invigorating.

I am confident that this book will offer the same sense of independence, achievement and help to those who read it.

1998   Carolyn Hicks

Preface

I teach statistics to health studies students, undergraduate nurses, and a mixture of nurses, physiotherapists, podiatrists and other health professionals at Masters level. For the undergraduates I have no problems in finding texts. Most nursing research textbooks have a section on basic statistics, for example.[1,2] For a slightly fuller (although at a similar level) introduction to statistics there are many excellent texts, particular favourites of my students being the two books by my colleague Dr Carolyn Hicks (who wrote the foreword to this book).[3,4]

However, when you move from basic statistics to even an intermediate level, the texts designed for health care professionals are few, and mainly directed towards psychology rather than nursing or the professions allied to medicine (e.g. physiotherapy, podiatry and occupational therapy). There are many excellent texts covering all the statistical methods any health care professional would care to use, but these are typically written with professions other than health care, such as engineering, business or economics, in mind. I have found that, while the content and style of many such texts are excellent, my students cannot transfer the concepts to their area – they need examples drawn from health care. Furthermore, to cover all the statistics, the students will need several texts.

As I have failed to identify any single text I could recommend to my students, I have written this one. This book will be suitable for students undertaking more advanced courses, or who have specific statistical requirements for their dissertations. Typical readers might be final year undergraduates in nursing or one of the professions allied to medicine, taught Masters students, or health workers performing research as part of their clinical duties.

1998   Denis Anthony

REFERENCES

1. Dempsey P A, Dempsey A D 1996 Nursing research: text and workbook. Little, Brown, Boston
2. Clifford C 1997 Nursing & health care research. Prentice Hall, London
3. Hicks C M 1988 Practical research methods for physiotherapists. Churchill Livingstone, Edinburgh
4. Hicks C M 1990 Research and statistics: a practical introduction for nurses. Prentice Hall, Heme

Acknowledgements

The author is indebted to the following: Dr Mike Clarke, of Pegasus Airwave Systems, and Ms Frances Healey, of York District General Hospital, for allowing access to pressure-sore assessment data on inpatients; Ms Victoria Naughten, one of my nursing students, who had the original idea of considering differences in branch examination scores, and permitted me to present the statistics suggested in her research proposal; Dr Jim Unsworth, of the West Midlands Rehabilitation Service, for allowing access to pressure-sore assessment data on wheelchair users; the various reviewers of the chapters; and the staff of Churchill Livingstone who offered helpful advice and improved the content and presentation of the material.

1

Introduction

I have identified several statistical methods that are commonly employed in health care journals, especially of the more academic sort, that are either not covered at all, or only in insufficient detail, in basic texts dealing with health care statistics. A review of statistics used in the *Journal of Advanced Nursing*, for example, showed that of 45 papers that had any statistical content in 6 months of 1994, the statistical tests listed in Table 1.1 were found on at least two occasions.[1]

These tests, being the common ones in the academic press, should be included in a complete text. Of these tests, those that compare means (Student's *t*-test) or distributions (Mann–Whitney) are well covered in basic texts, but extensions into more than two groups, using ANOVA or Kruskall–Wallis, for example, would probably not be mentioned in simpler texts. Correlation using the Spearman rank or Pearson tests are usually adequately covered in basic texts, but many methods employing

Table 1.1 Survey of statistical tests used in 45 papers in *Journal of Advanced Nursing* (1994)

Test	No.	% of total articles
Chi square (χ^2)	14	31.1
Mann–Whitney	9	20.0
Analysis of variance (ANOVA)	7	15.6
Cronbach alpha (α)	7	15.6
Student's *t*-test (independent)	6	13.3
Factor analysis	4	8.9
Kruskall–Wallis	3	6.7
Spearman rank	3	6.7
Pearson	3	6.7
Student's *t*-test (paired)	2	4.4
Kappa (κ)	2	4.4

correlation, such as factor analysis, are only covered in more advanced books, and these are generally not aimed at health care workers.

This book is not intended to cover all statistics that a health care worker would need. There would be no point to this, as the simpler texts already available are both very readable and cover much of the material needed; furthermore, they are available in cheap editions. However, the intermediate material is rarely covered, and never in any depth, in basic statistics or research books for health care workers. The tests listed as common in nursing (the largest sector), and not dissimilar to other professions allied to medicine (PAM) are:

- *Comparisons of more than two groups.* For parametric testing this will be analysis of variance (ANOVA). ANOVA is a very powerful technique, and can be used in both independent groups and for repeated measures.
- *Measures of reliability,* such as agreement between observers (Cohen's κ) or measures of internal reliability for groups of variables (split half or Cronbach's α).
- *Methods using correlation as a basis.* Regression, where predictions of one or more dependent variables are made from one or more independent variables, is one example. Another is factor analysis (FA) and principal-components analysis (PCA), where a dataset is reduced to its most important elements.
- *Cluster analysis,* where groups of cases that are 'similar' to each other are arranged into some form or hierarchy or taxonomy.
- *Contingency tables.* Although the most well known use of contingency tables (χ^2) is covered in almost all texts, there are a variety of other, often as simple, tests that use nominal variables in contingency tables. For example, tests of association, and the assessment of relative risk.

However, a text that looked to the current literature only would not be advancing statistical practice in health care, but rather would merely be recording the correct use of those already in the literature. While I see the latter as one purpose of this book, there is a second one I wish to pursue. I believe that many statistical methods that would be most beneficial in nursing and PAM, are not employed because they are not known about.

Methods that are well known in other disciplines (medicine, psychology and medical physics) but barely used, if used at all, in the target group of this text are:

- *Receiver operating characteristic (ROC).* This method assesses the sensitivity and specificity of a scoring system at a variety of different scores. It is needed to compare two classification systems. An example given in this book is of different risk assessment scores for decubitus ulcer.
- *Artificial neural networks (ANNs).* These are computer programs that attempt to mimic the human brain (in a very crude fashion) to allow the

formation of concepts that are generalizable. Patterns are recognized rather than analysed. A typical application would be to 'train' the ANN using many examples of diseased and normal electrocardiogram (ECG; EKG in the USA) readings. After training, the ANN would hopefully correctly pick out the abnormal from the normal in new (unseen) readings.

Finally, there are areas that are of vital importance in designing or interpreting statistics, that seem surprisingly absent, even in intermediate and advanced texts:

• *Errors in the use of statistics*. Typically these are errors of omission, such as failure to state the type of test used. However, there are some very common errors of commission, such as the inappropriate use of parametric tests on obviously non-normal data.
• *Power analysis*. This addresses the question of how many subjects are needed in order to get a meaningful result.

This book therefore attempts to cover four main areas:

1. The use of statistics a little more advanced than that covered in basic research and statistics texts aimed at nursing, physiotherapy and other PAM. This material is mainstream in that it commonly appears in articles in the academic journals read by these professional groups.
2. The introduction of techniques that are rarely or never used in academic articles by nurses and the PAM, but which I believe are of great potential in aiding some types of enquiry in these fields.
3. A discussion of the errors in reporting statistics.
4. An introduction to the scientific approach to identifying the numbers needed in your study.

CONCEPTS BASIC TO THIS TEXT

Data types

Data are said to be of four levels:

• *Nominal*: data that are categorical; they can be coded into numbers, but these numbers would simply be labels. An example would be gender, which can be male (coded 1, say) or female (coded 2, say), but females are not twice males.
• *Ordinal*: data that have an inherent ordering; for example, the position in a race (first, second, third, etc.). The numbers show position, but we do not know the size of the intervals between first and second, or whether it is different to that between second and third.
• *Interval*: data where intervals are the same between 1 and 2, 2 and 3,

etc. Temperature centigrade is an example, where the difference between 36°C and 37°C is precisely one degree, and it is not merely the case that 37°C is higher than 36°C.

- *Ratio*: interval data that, in addition, have an absolute zero. For example, an object cannot have less than zero weight, while an object that weighs 60 kg is exactly twice the weight of a 30 kg object. In contradistinction, a temperature of 40°C is not twice that of 20°C, and it is possible to have a temperature less than zero.

There is a hierarchy of data types: the ratio type subsumes the other three (i.e. ratio data are also interval, ordinal and nominal data); interval data are also ordinal and nominal; and ordinal data are also nominal. However, we refer to data by the highest level at which they exist. Statistical tests that are suitable for use on nominal data may not be (and usually are not) optimal for higher data types. Statistical tests can be split into three types: those that are used on nominal data (χ^2, for example), those used on ordinal data (Mann–Whitney, for example), and those that are used on interval/ratio data (Student's t-test, for example, although some authors recommend its use on ordinal data if the data are normally distributed).

p value

In all inferential statistics a p value is given. This is the probability that the results found could have occurred by chance alone. This is measured on a scale of 0–1, so $p = 0.05$ means 5%, or a 1 in 20 chance, and $p = 0.01$ means a 1%, or 1 in 100 chance. A common error is to assume that a high p value means that the result is significant; in fact, a *low* value shows significance.

Type I error

The possibility of obtaining the results by chance alone is indicated by the p value. But, however small the value of p may be, there is always a finite chance that the results were purely due to chance, and any apparent differences between group means (for example) are pure artefact. A p value of 0.05 means that 1 time in 20 you could expect such a result by chance. The occasions where the data did in fact occur due to chance can be considered to be in error if the p value is accepted as showing a real difference (in the case of two mean values). This is known as a type I error. You can reduce type I error to any level you care to define. For example, if you considered it problematic to accept type I errors 5% of the time, but could accept them 1% of the time, you would only accept p values under 0.01 as being significant.

Type II error

This is the opposite of type I error, and is seen when you accept that the results were due to chance, when in fact this is not true. For example, a small correlation between two variables might be given a p value of 0.03, which means that 3% of the time it could have occurred by chance alone. If we used a threshold for the p value under 0.05 to mean the result was unlikely to have occurred by chance, we would in this case (correctly) reject the null hypothesis. However, if as above for the type I error, we considered this not stringent enough and only reject the null hypothesis if the p value is under 0.01, then we consider this to be not low enough to be sure, and (incorrectly in this case) accept the null hypothesis. Clearly, the lower we set the threshold at which we reject the null hypothesis the more likely are type II errors.

α value

A low p value is said to be significant, but how low? This is a matter of compromise, as giving a low threshold for a p value which we will consider significant will increase type II errors, and raising the threshold will increase type I errors. Conventionally a threshold (called the α value) is set at 0.05, so any value under 0.05 is considered to be significant, and any value equal to or above 0.05 is considered not significant. However, there are many authors (me, for example) who see no real difference between a p value of 0.049 and one of 0.051, the former of which would be considered significant and the latter not, by the criterion of using an α value of 0.05. An alternative to using a rigid α value is to quote all probabilities and allow the reader to decide what is significant.

Parametric and non-parametric tests

Any statistical test makes some assumptions about the data. A group of tests, so called *parametric tests*, assume the data are *normally distributed*, i.e. the histogram of values shows a bell-shaped curve, with most values lying close to the middle of the distribution, and increasingly extreme values seen with increasingly lower frequency. However, not all data are normal, and then these tests should not be applied (in most cases), but an equivalent non-parametric test, which does not assume a normal distribution, is to be preferred.

This book concentrates on parametric tests, but in most cases an equivalent non-parametric test is available, and does a similar job.

CONCLUSION

I have identified why I believe this book is needed, and what it will cover.

Most inferential statistical tests (on which this book concentrates) can be described as one of two broad types:

- Tests assessing the significance of differences between groups. These include the parametric tests Student's t-test, for two groups, and analysis of variance (ANOVA), for more than two groups. ANOVA is covered in Chapter 6.
- Tests of correlation among two or more variables. Correlation, which is covered in Chapter 4, shows how much one variable can be accounted for by another variable, or by several other variables. Correlation is the basis for other more powerful techniques, such as regression, FA and PCA, which are described in Chapter 9.

REFERENCES

1. Anthony D M 1996 A review of statistical methods in the *Journal of Advanced Nursing*. Journal of Advanced Nursing 24: 1089–1094.

2

Introduction to SPSS for Windows

SPSS is a powerful statistics system. It is the computer package on which this book is based. This chapter introduces the reader to the interface, 'look and feel' and some of the basic features of the system.

KEY POINTS

- SPSS runs under the most common operating systems, Microsoft Windows 95 and Windows 3.11 under MS-DOS, as well as other mainframe and microcomputer systems
- Originally designed for the social sciences, SPSS is a mature product, and has many modules to cater for most statistics applications. It is one of the main statistics packages available, other systems include SAS, BMDP, Statview and Minitab.
- SPSS is able to create graphs as well as compute statistics
- In addition to many reference works on SPSS, there is a tutorial guide available on the system

At the end of this chapter the student should be able to:

1. Start SPSS from Windows

7

2. Create a new or open an existing SPSS file

3. Define and change variables

4. Perform simple statistics

5. Create a simple graph

6. Quit SPSS

INTRODUCTION

The Statistical Package for the Social Sciences (SPSS, which is a trademark of SPSS Inc., Chicago, IL, USA)[1,3] is one of the most popular and most powerful statistics software packages available. There are other similarly powerful packages, for example SAS (SAS is a trademark of SAS Institute Inc., Cary, NC, USA)[2] or BMDP,[4] but in my opinion the interface of SPSS, though by no means ideal, is superior to the others I have tried. There are other smaller and possibly easier packages to use, such as StatView[5] and Minitab,[6] but these are not as flexible or as powerful, features that are increasingly needed as more advanced statistics are used.

SPSS runs on a variety of systems, for example UNIX, MS-DOS (Microsoft), Windows (Windows is a trademark of Microsoft Inc., Seattle, WA, USA) and the Macintosh (Apple Computers Inc., San Francisco, CA, USA) operating system. Here we look at the most common system, Windows. The version of SPSS running under Windows is simply called SPSS for Windows.

MICROSOFT WINDOWS

Older computing systems required the user to type in commands via a keyboard. Many potential users found this difficult, and computer usage for this and many other reasons (e.g. cost of computers) restricted usage of computers to technically minded people such as engineers and computer scientists.

In the 1980s after research on interfaces initiated by Xerox, the Macintosh computer interface was developed, which showed most computer functions as icons that resembled the task which they should perform, and made extensive use of the mouse rather than typed commands. For example, to delete a file you would drag the icon representing the file to an icon of a waste-paper basket.

Microsoft later developed their own graphics system to supersede MS-DOS, and called it simply Windows. Figure 2.1 shows the Windows interface for Windows 3.11 (there are several versions of Windows, the current most common for personal use are Windows 3.11 and Windows '95).

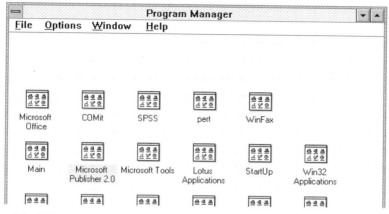

Figure 2.1 Windows 3.11 Program Manager.

Windows 3.11

The Program Manager is the utility (or program) that controls all the other programs (which could include word processors, spreadsheet programs, etc.) and it shows the other programs as icons to make them as small as possible on the screen, and gives them labels so you know what they are. For example, SPSS is shown as the third item on the top row. The exact look of the screen you will use may be different, as you may have different programs on your system.

If you double click ('click' in this text means depress the left mouse key once, 'double click' means depress the left mouse key twice in quick succession) on the icon it opens out into a *window* (Fig. 2.2). If you are new to using a mouse you may find it easier to click on the word 'window', the third word from the left at the top of the screen, and from the pull-down menu choose SPSS.

In this new SPSS window, which overlays the Program Manager window, you see several new icons, including a tutorial guide to SPSS, but the one you select to run the actual statistics package is the one simply entitled 'SPSS' (the actual style of the icons you see may vary according to the version of SPSS for Windows you possess). If you double click on the SPSS icon, the SPSS program will start.

Windows '95

Windows '95 is (at the time of writing) the most recent Windows interface. If you are using this interface, then all programs may be started by clicking on the Start button, which is normally located at the bottom left-hand corner of the screen. This will bring up a *pop-up menu*, from which

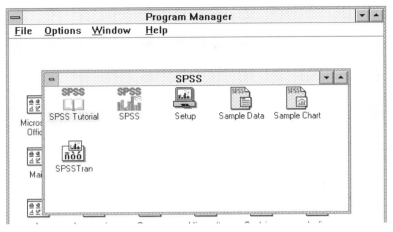

Figure 2.2   The SPSS window and icons.

you can select items by clicking on the relevant item. Click on Programs and another pop-up menu appears; select SPSS and a final pop-up menu appears with all the SPSS programs (in addition to the statistics program there is a tutorial guide and other utilities), from which you should select SPSS again.

RUNNING SPSS FOR WINDOWS

Once you are running SPSS for Windows, the behaviour is much the same whichever version of Windows you are using, with the exception that re-sizing the windows, and some other common operations that are nothing to do with the packages as such, are slightly different.

Figure 2.3 shows SPSS as it appears when you first run it. This (and most other figures in this text) show the Windows 3.11 interface, which is the one I use, as the Windows '95 interface seems less robust to me. If you are using Windows '95 the main difference is that the top right-hand corner of each window contains three small icons, whereas the 3.11 version contains two (an up arrow and a down arrow, as shown in Fig. 2.2).

On entry, SPSS shows three windows: the main SPSS window; and two subwindows within SPSS, the Newdata and Output windows (the former overlies the latter almost entirely).

Windows 3.11

If you click on the down arrow (the left of the two arrows at the top right of the SPSS screen) in the main SPSS window it will disappear and an icon called SPSS will be seen on the screen within the program manager. If you

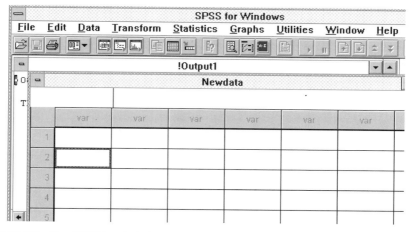

Figure 2.3 The SPSS input window.

double click on the icon SPSS, the SPSS main window (and its associated subwindows) will reappear. If you click on the down arrow in any particular subwindow, it will disappear and become an icon in the main SPSS window; you can get it back by double clicking on the icon.

If you click on the up arrow of any window (next to the down arrow), the window will become as large as it can (if the up arrow of the main SPSS window is clicked, the window fills the screen; if one of the SPSS subwindows is used it will fill the entire space of the original SPSS main window, totally obscuring it). There will now be a new symbol, a double arrow (pointing both up and down); if this symbol is clicked, then the window will return to its original size.

Windows '95

If you click on the flat line (the left of the three icons at the top right of the SPSS screen) in the main SPSS window, the window will disappear and the title SPSS will be seen at the bottom of the screen in the *title bar*. If you double click on the title SPSS, the main window (and its associated subwindows) will reappear. If you click on the flat line icon in any particular subwindow, that subwindow will disappear and become a title in the title bar of the main SPSS window; you can get it back by double clicking on the title.

If you click on the square icon of any window (next to the flat line icon), the window will become as large as it can (if the flat line icon of the main SPSS window is clicked, the window fills the screen; if one of the SPSS subwindows is used, it will fill the entire space of the original SPSS main window, totally obscuring it). There will now be a new symbol, a square within a square; if this symbol is clicked the window will return to its original size.

The rightmost icon is a cross (X). This is used to 'kill' a program (i.e. terminate or finish running that program). If you click on this by accident you will usually be asked to confirm that you do really want to leave the program. It is not typically the best way to terminate a program.

On either Windows 3.11 or '95

Thus you can have any window totally filling the screen, or filling only a portion of the screen, or an icon merely showing that the window exists. It is important to realize that the iconified program is still running, and any data, graphs, etc., you may create will still be there when you de-iconify it (i.e. when you double click on the icon to make it a window again).

As an alternative to using the mouse, for any menu item there should be a 'hot key', which allows you to select the menu, submenu or item of a menu from the keyboard. This is done by holding down the 'Alt' key (often found to the left of the spacebar) and, while it is held down, hitting briefly a given key of the keyboard. The given key will be underlined in the menu item; for example, to activate the File menu in SPSS, you use Alt+F (the Alt key held down, with the F key hit briefly).

If you have difficulty with the mouse, you can use the keyboard instead for all operations. For example, in the Program Manager Alt+W will get the Windows pull-down menu, and using the down or up arrow key allows you to select the package (SPSS in this case), which is shown as selected with a tick. Hitting the Return key will open the SPSS window, and using the left and right arrow keys you can select the program (SPSS in this case), which is run when you hit the Return key.

OPENING AN EXISTING FILE

You can retrieve previously stored data files in order to carry on working on data. If you click the File menu item at the top left of the main window, a pull-down menu appears (Fig. 2.4). Note that in Figure 2.4 SPSS may not be taking up the whole screen, and some other icons and programs may be partly visible underneath the SPSS window; these are nothing to do with SPSS. For example a printer icon and a word processing program icon, which are running at the same time as SPSS, could be shown. This shows a feature of Windows, that many things can be run at the same time. The screen is visually two dimensional, but you should think of it as three dimensional, with other programs possibly 'hiding' behind the current window.

To open a file, the Open item is selected with the left mouse button (or using Alt+O, note the letter 'oh', *not* zero). You are then given the option of opening several different types of file (see Fig. 2.4), including data files.

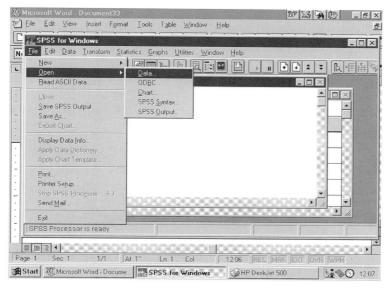

Figure 2.4   Opening an existing data file.

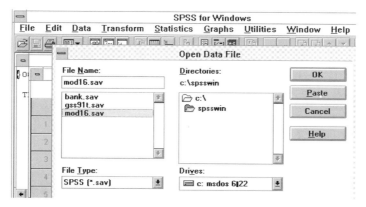

Figure 2.5   Dialogue box for opening a data file.

Selecting Data brings up a *dialogue box*, as shown in Figure 2.5. A dialogue box is where you can enter information that does not fit the rigidity of menus. Here you see you can select a file (there are three shown). The file selected in the figure (by clicking on the file name) is mod16.sav. SPSS data files, by default, have the ending (suffix) '.sav', which indicates an SPSS data file as opposed to, for example, a graphics file from SPSS or a file from some other package (e.g. Word for Windows, the word processing package).

It is possible, indeed likely, that you will want to keep your data files in

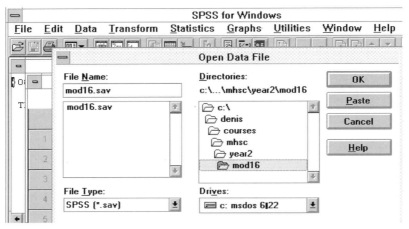

Figure 2.6   Opening a data file in a different directory.

a different directory to the one SPSS assumes (typically 'spsswin', but this depends on how the package was installed). Directories are like filing cabinets where files of a similar type may be kept. Figure 2.6 shows how you can select a different directory. This was done by clicking on the item c:\ under Directories in the centre of the screen, and then selecting in turn 'denis', courses, mhsc, year2 and, finally, mod16. This shows a nested directory structure, where groups of directories themselves are in a higher level directory. That is, I have all my module 16 files in a directory called mod16, and these are combined with other modules into the second year of a Masters course in the directory year2, which is in mhsc with other years, and all courses are likewise placed together under my personal directory called 'denis'.

Your file store will have a different structure to the one shown in Figure 2.6, but may also have nested directories so that you can find files more easily. You may not want as deep a nesting as I use, but putting all files in the same place is asking for trouble (imagine finding one letter from a single pile on your desk where you have stored all correspondence from the last 2 years). Directories and subdirectories (directories within directories) are created outside of SPSS: in Windows 3.11 you use the File Manager, which is part of the 'main' window (see Fig. 2.1); and in Windows '95 you can use the My Computer icon, or the File Manager under Programs.

Having selected the file, in this case mod16.sav, the data will be displayed in the input window (Fig. 2.7).

CREATING A NEW FILE

To create a totally new file, from the File menu, select New, then Data (Fig.

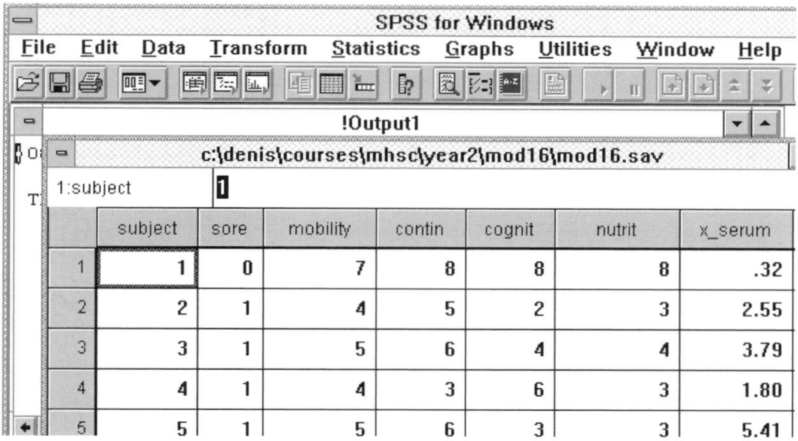

Figure 2.7   A data input window.

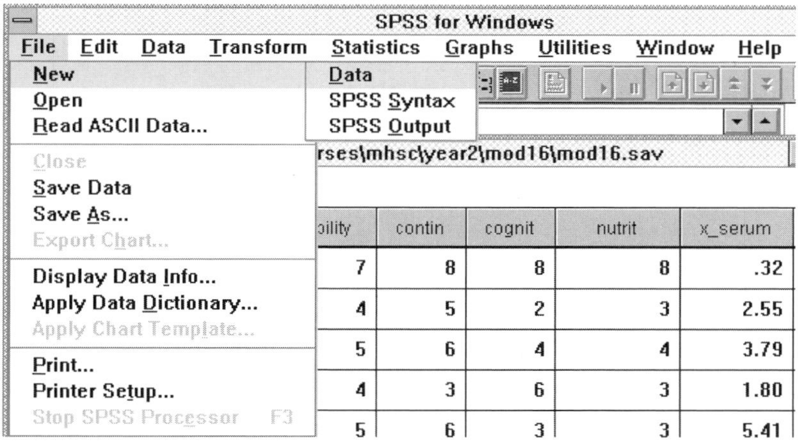

Figure 2.8   Creating a new data file.

2.8) and then hit the Return key (or double click on the left mouse button). A completely empty data window appears (Fig. 2.9). If you enter data, say the number '1', in the first cell of the data window, initially the number appears above the data cells, but when you hit the return key it will be placed in the first cell (Fig. 2.10). You can move to different data cells by clicking the mouse in a cell, or by using the arrow keys on the keyboard (typically located on the right of the keyboard). When the data extend to more than the window can show, you can use the scroll bars (on the right and bottom edges of the window) or the Page Up and Page Down keys on

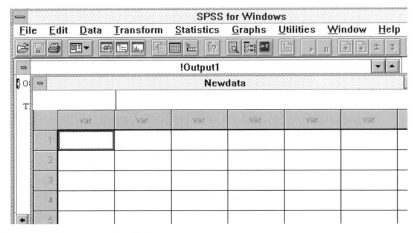

Figure 2.9   A new data file window.

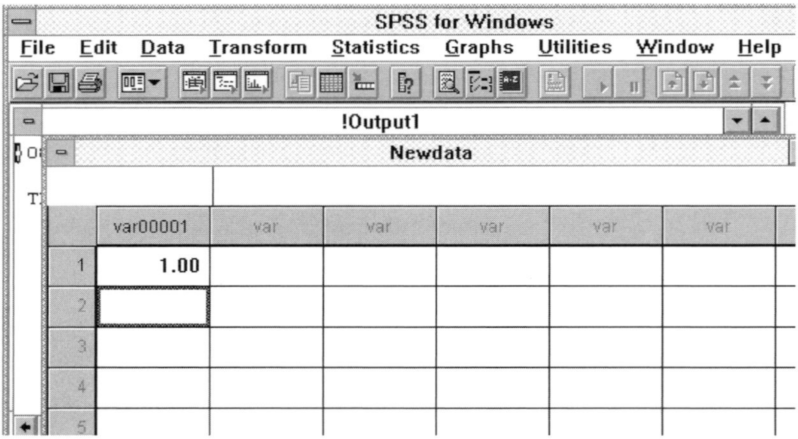

Figure 2.10   Entering data in the data window.

the keyboard. Scroll bars can be used by clicking on the arrows (left and right arrows at either end of the horizontal bar, and up and down arrows on the vertical bar), or by 'grabbing' the small square that indicates the current position on the scroll bar by clicking the mouse button on the square, holding the button down and dragging it.

RENAMING THE VARIABLES

SPSS arranges data as rows and columns. Rows are subjects (often people) and columns are variables recorded on each subject. So row 1 might be for a patient in a study, with subsequent rows being for more subjects in the same study, and column 1 might contain the age of each subject.

When SPSS starts a new file there are no data and no variable names. As soon as data are entered in any column, that column is given a data variable name, something like 'var00001'. This is necessary, as you need to be able to refer to the variable name later, but is not very memorable as a name.

If you double click on the variable name (or on the menu click on Data and then on Define Variable), the Define Variable dialogue box appears (Fig. 2.11). You can change the name of the variable; here I will choose 'age' by simply typing 'age' using the keyboard.

Changing the data type

There are many options when defining the variable. If you select Type, the new dialogue box shown in Figure 2.12 will be shown. Note I have changed the variable name already.

SPSS allows many data types, but the most common is Numeric, which has a given number of decimal places and overall length; by default, this is a width of eight and two decimal places, so the largest number it will show is 99999.99 (eight digits long, including the decimal place). However, age is not typically given to this accuracy, or able to reach this size. A better choice for age would probably be zero decimal places and a length of three (i.e. any number up to 999, with no decimal points allowed).

If an item of data is entered that is not within the number of digits chosen, it will be shown as asterisks; alternatively, if the entry has more

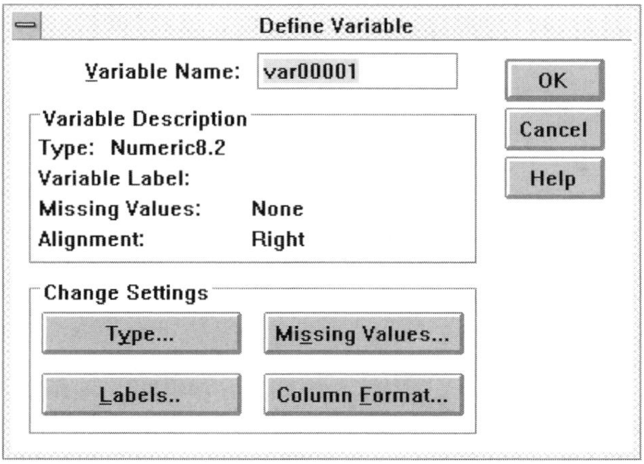

Figure 2.11   Defining a variable.

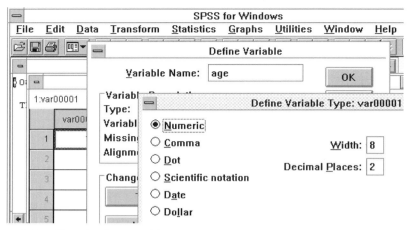

Figure 2.12 Changing the type of data.

decimal places than specified, the extra decimals will not be shown. However, the number entered will not be lost, it is simply not shown, to indicate that the number is probably wrong. When you are in a specific cell, the real value contained within it is shown on the top of the input window, and if you change the settings for the size of the number, the full number will be shown in the cell if it is now within the new defined number range.

Labelling the data

Looking again at Figure 2.11, there is also a Labels option. The variable name is restricted to eight digits and must not contain spaces, but a longer *label* can be applied to the variable (Fig. 2.13). Each value of the variable can also be labelled. This is only useful if the data are nominal or ordinal. Gender, for example, can be denoted by numbers, such as 1 for female and 2 for male (for speed of data entry). These numbers can be labelled, so that at a later date you will know what they signify. Also, any graphs or statistics output will show the label rather than the actual value, so a pie chart would show 'female' rather than '1'.

SIMPLE STATISTICS

About the simplest statistics that can be computed are frequencies. The Statistics pull-down menu is obtained by clicking on the fifth from the left (Fig. 2.14). Selecting Summarize from this menu gives another pull-down menu that includes Frequencies. Selecting this menu item gives you the

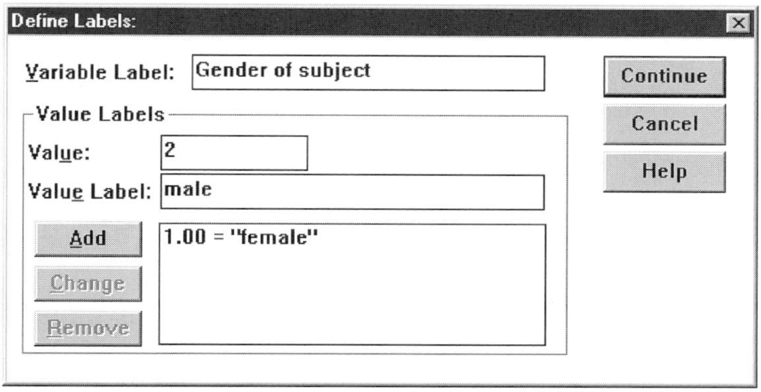

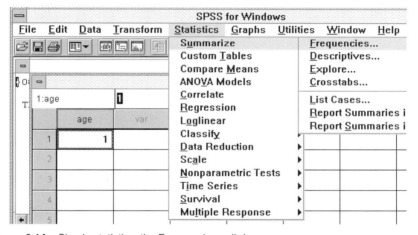

Figure 2.13   Data variable tables.

Figure 2.14   Simple statistics: the Frequencies pull-down menu.

dialogue box shown in Figure 2.15. By default the option gives you only the frequencies of a given variable, although there are many other possibilities. You can find out the frequencies of as many variables as you like, but in Figure 2.15 I have chosen just one variable, age. This was done by selecting the variable from the list of variables on the left, and then clicking the arrow. Having done this the arrow changes direction to allow you to move the variable back to the list if chosen by accident (this is the position we are at in Figure 2.15). If you select another variable on the left-hand list, the arrow changes direction to point to the right again. Many of the dialogue boxes in SPSS are like this; i.e. if one or more variables can be

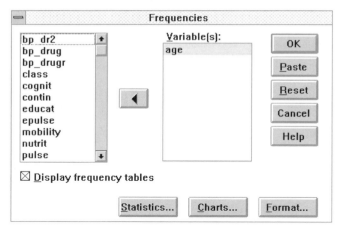

Figure 2.15 Simple statistics: the Frequencies dialogue box.

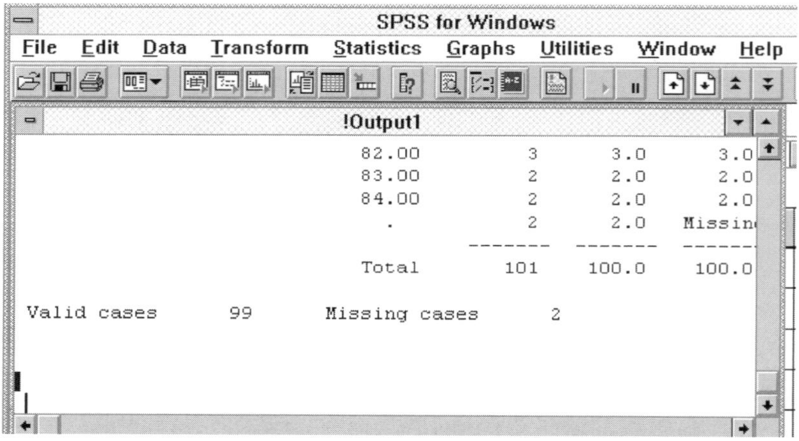

Figure 2.16 The Output window.

selected from a list, you can move the variable back again and/or select another.

Having chosen your variables, select the OK button and the output window is now created, overlying the input window (Fig. 2.16). The whole of the output cannot be seen in the output window, and you can scroll around using the scroll bars, or make the window full-screen size by using the 'up' arrow (Fig. 2.17) (note that the 'up' arrow is now replaced by the double arrow). You still can only see the bottom half of the table, so you should use the 'up' scroll bar or the Page Up key (possibly labelled PgUp on your keyboard) to see the top of the table.

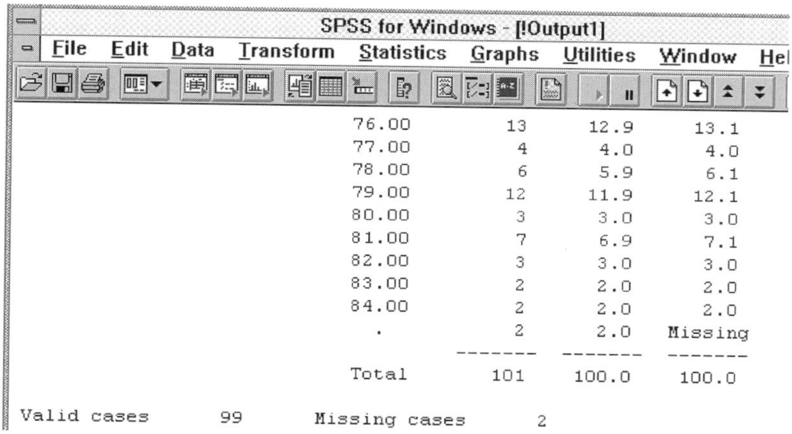

Figure 2.17   The Output window: full screen.

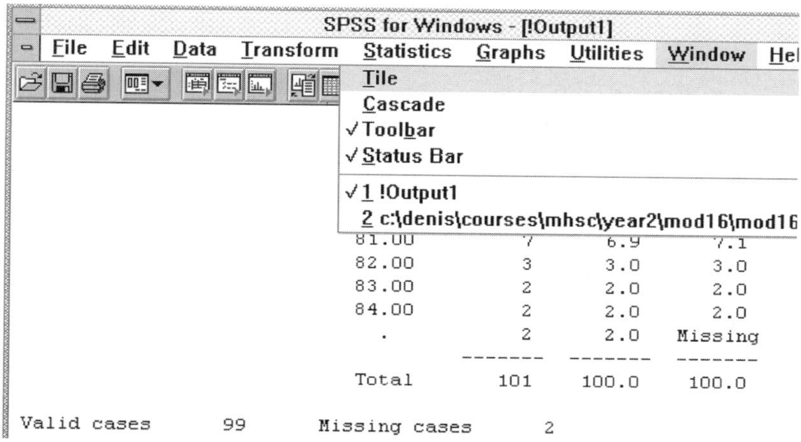

Figure 2.18   Finding 'lost' windows.

LOST WINDOWS

As mentioned above, Windows is conceptually three dimensional, but you can only see two-dimensional images on the screen. Therefore, a window may 'hide' another window that is behind it, and this can be confusing. You can always find lost windows by using the Window menu. Figure 2.18 shows the current windows, numbered 1 and 2. The current window (1) is ticked. If you click on '2' then that window (here the data window) will reappear.

GRAPHS

Graphs can be obtained via the Graphs pull-down menu (Fig. 2.19), which lists many different graphs. If you choose, say, Histogram, you will get the dialogue box shown in Figure 2.20. You can only have one variable for a histogram, and again I have chosen 'age'. Note that I have also elected to draw a normal curve (bottom centre of the box). After selecting OK, the histogram in Figure 2.21 is shown (it is noticeably non-normal).

If you iconify the graph (by clicking the 'down' arrow) the chart disappears to the icon Carousel, or in Windows '95 is minimised as shown in Figure 2.22 at the bottom left of the main SPSS window. Note we now have three

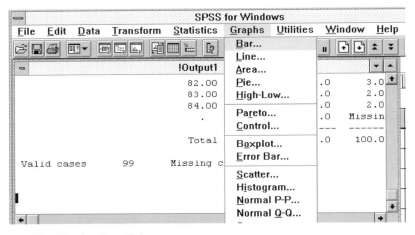

Figure 2.19 The Graphs pull-down menu.

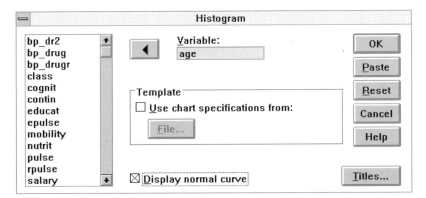

Figure 2.20 The Histogram dialogue box.

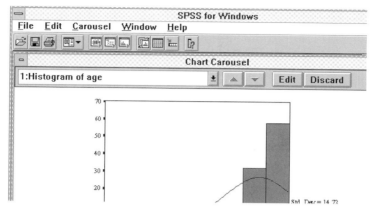

Figure 2.21   A histogram in the Chart Carousel.

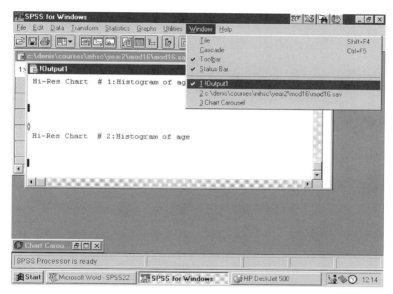

Figure 2.22   The Chart Carousel window minimised and the Windows pull-down menu.

windows, as shown with the Windows pull-down menu. You can get the graph back either by clicking on '3' in the Windows pull-down, or by double clicking the Carousel icon.

As with many other aspects of SPSS, there are many ways of achieving the same ends. In this case you could have got the same histogram from the Frequencies item of the Statistics menu. Looking at Figure 2.15 you will see the Charts option, which contains an option for producing exactly the same histogram. Try it!

WHERE DO I GO FROM HERE?

Although you can read the SPSS manual, this is often not the best way to get further help. In many cases the online hypertext Windows help facility is more useful. In nearly all Windows programs (also called *applications*) the help facility is called up by hitting the function key F1 or by clicking on the Help pull-down (rightmost menu pull-down; see e.g. Fig. 2.22).

The SPSS online help is extensive. You can go through it, like a textbook, by going through the contents. Hypertext systems such as the Windows help facility have *links*, which are shown in Figure 2.23 as underlined phrases. If you click on a link you will be taken to that part of the online manual.

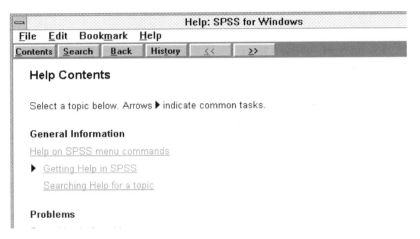

Figure 2.23   The Help hypertext system.

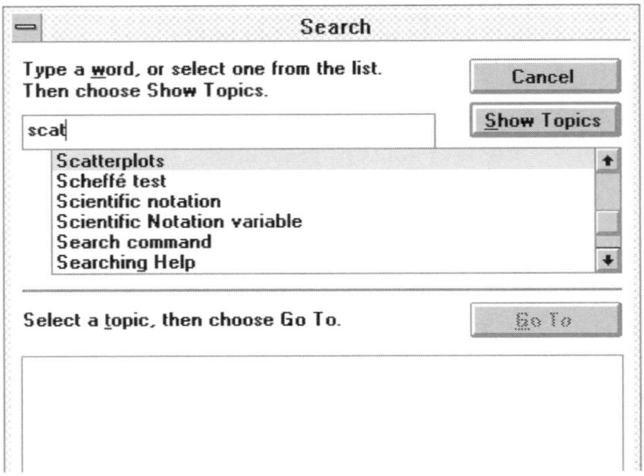

Figure 2.24   The Search help facility.

An alternative way to get help is to use the Search facility (Fig. 2.24). As you type in a phrase the Help facility tries to match your request. For example, when looking for 'scatterplot' I had to type only the first four letters before a match was found. Clicking on Show Topics then gives the dialogue box shown in Figure 2.25, where it can be seen that several parts of the online manual are about scatterplots. As I am interested in charts, I select that topic (by double clicking, or pressing the Return key) and this gives me Figure 2.26, which you will note also has hypertext links (e.g. if you click on the icon at the top left of the page, you will be shown where the scatterplot is located in the menu pull-downs).

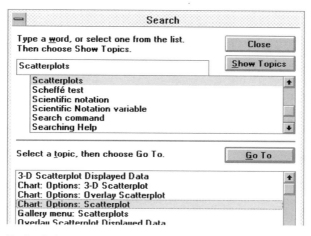

Figure 2.25   Finding help on scatterplots.

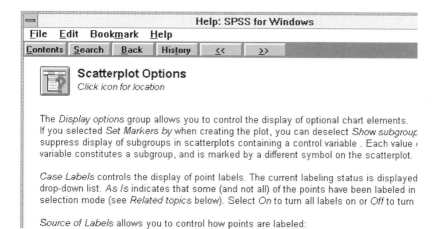

Figure 2.26   The scatterplot help page.

The SPSS manuals are many in number, each one several hundred pages long, and it is not the purpose of this text to show every aspect of SPSS. However, you should by now have the 'look and feel' of the software in that new dialogue boxes are all pretty similar to ones shown above, and by using the online help facility you can learn as you go.

SPSS also has an online tutorial (see Fig. 2.2). If you are still having difficulties, try running this instead of the SPSS package when you open the SPSS window.

LEAVING SPSS

Click on File and then select Exit (see Fig. 2.4). If you have not saved your files you will be asked if you want to do so. In most cases you only need to save the data, as graphs and output can always be re-created from the data. Sometimes it is helpful to save charts and output (especially the former, if a lot of work has been put into customizing a graph for a report, for example).

EXERCISES

1. Run SPSS by selecting the appropriate icon or menu option from Windows or Windows '95.

2. Define two new variables called 'Waterlow' and 'Sore'. These will be the Waterlow scores (a scale of risk where scores higher than 10 mean the patient is at risk) for patients who may or may not have pressure sores.

3. Enter the data given in the table below into the two new variables.

Waterlow score	21.00	17.00	14.00	19.00	31.00	22.00	4.00	19.00	17.00	9.00	13.00
Sore	1	1	0	0	1	0	0	0	1	0	1

4. Change the variable 'sore' so that it does not show decimal points (hint use Type from Define Variable).

5. Make a further change to 'sore' by adding two labels that identify 0 as normal (no sore), and 1 as being a sore (hint use Lables from Define Variable).

6. Compute the number of patients with sores by using Statistics then Summarize then Frequencies.

7. Using Graphs, create a pie chart showing the proportion of patients with sores and the proportion of normal patients.

8. Using Graphs again, create a frequency histogram of Waterlow scores.

REFERENCES

1. Norusis M J 1993 SPSS for Windows base system user's guide. SPSS, Chicago, IL
2. SAS Institute Inc. 1982 SAS users' guide: statistics. SAS Institute Inc., Cary, NC
3. SPSS Inc. 1983 SPSS-X users' guide. McGraw-Hill, New York
4. Dixon W J, Wilfred J (eds) 1981 BMDP Statistical software manual. University of California Press, Berkeley, CA
5. Abacus Concepts 1992 Statview. Abacus Concepts, Berkeley, CA 300–319
6. Ryan B F, Joiner B L, Ryan T A 1995 Minitab. Duxbury Press, Boston, MA

Validity and reliability

Validity is a measure of relevance, and reliability measures the stability of a study. They are quite distinct attributes. A highly valid study is one that addresses the area of interest; such a study may or may not be repeatable. A reliable study will give similar results when it is repeated, but this does not necessarily imply that it is of any relevance. This chapter looks at some methods to ensure valid and reliable studies.

KEY POINTS

- Validity addresses the appropriateness or relevance of measurements
- Reliability measures how repeatable measures are
- Reliability is not synonymous with accuracy
- Measures of agreement need to account for the agreement expected by chance
- Internal reliability measures the extent to which components of a research tool (typically a questionnaire) are measuring the same thing

At the end of this chapter the student should be able to:

1. Identify methods of ensuring validity of measurements or research tools used

2. State what measures of reliability are appropriate for a given set of data

3. Set up SPSS to measure internal and external reliability

4. Interpret the output from SPSS for internal and external reliability

INTRODUCTION

Validity and reliability are highly important, though often overlooked, aspects of any study, whether quantitative (inferential or descriptive) or qualitative. *Validity* refers to whether you are measuring, recording, observing or assessing the appropriate items; in other words, are the data relevant? *Reliability* is a measure of how repeatable the data are that are captured; i.e. if I do this experiment again will I get the same value for blood sugar, or if I interview the same person twice will their answers be similar or both occasions?

It is possible to get highly repeatable results that are inaccurate, for example if my weighing scale is weighing consistently light it may always report me a kilogram below my real weight, although it may be always within 0.1 kg of the previous reading. A less reliable scale (say consecutive readings within 0.2 kg of each other) may be more accurate, with a mean value close to my real weight. So reliability is not the same as *accuracy*. However, if you always use the same instrument, the fact that it is reliable may be more useful than its accuracy. If I want to lose weight the scales that are always one kilogram too low will still allow me to see if I am losing or gaining. Paradoxically, these inaccurate scales are more useful than the more accurate but less reliable ones, provided I always use the same scales.

A highly reliable measuring device may not be a valid one. A micrometer is capable of measuring very tiny distances (thousandths of an inch), but this is of no use if you want to measure the length of a football pitch. Investigators sometimes choose highly accurate and/or highly reliable measures (remembering that accuracy and reliability are separate features) rather than less precise and/or less reliable measures that are actually relevant.

It is said of economists that they would rather be precisely wrong than roughly correct. If you wanted to measure poverty, an economist might suggest you could collect data on income, which may be available and be both reliable and accurate. However, while highly relevant to poverty, income is not the full story. Two people on the same income could be in very different positions. One might be in an area that has much cheaper living costs for example. A sociologist might suggest you consider how many items, considered by a set of focus groups to be indicative of poverty, a group of people possesses. Various such alternative measures of poverty that are not purely based on raw income have been suggested (another is a subsistence measure, i.e. whether a person can afford a basket of necessary foodstuffs; and another is a relative measure based on half or some fraction of the median income). All these measures have problems but, arguably, most or all of them are more valid than simply counting income.

Validity is the determination of the extent to which an instrument actually reflects the (often abstract) construct being examined, and *reliability* is how consistently an instrument (possibly a human observer) measures the concept of interest.

VALIDITY

There are several 'common sense' methods of dealing with validity. The way in which validity is defined varies between the texts. For example, Dempsey & Dempsey[1] have identified three types of validity:

- *Content validity.* In surveys, interviews or questionnaires, content validity is often used. Content validity is where each item is examined to see whether it is relevant, often by reference to the literature or previous studies. One method of achieving content validity is to ask experts in the field to examine the items. *Face validity* is a subset of content validity, where an item appears a priori to be sensible for inclusion in, say, a questionnaire. When making such a decision you are using your own knowledge and experience or that of some external assessor. Thus this method is not time consuming; but neither is it very rigorous. The use of pilot studies is mainly designed to address content validity. If a question is ambiguous or misunderstood, the answers obtained in the study will not be useful. A pilot study will typically pick up most of the serious problems in comprehension of an instrument.
- *Construct validity.* This is where the ability to measure some trait is assessed. If, for example, the intelligence of students studying for a doctorate compared with that of students who failed to obtain university entry did not differ according to some new scale of intelligence, then you might suspect that the scale was not valid. Factor analysis (see Ch. 9) may be used to create constructs from collections of variables.
- *Criterion-related validity.* This refers to how well a new instrument compares with some well tried older measure. For example, how does the Waterlow score for decubitus ulcer assessment compare with the Norton score? Since the latter is known to predict sores in a probabilistic fashion, a total lack of agreement between the scores would indicate that the Waterlow score would not be likely to be valid (as it happens, the two scores are very similar).

Bryman & Cramer[2] discuss validity in slightly different terms. They consider it to be composed of:

- *Face validity*. Defined as above.
- *Construct validity*. Defined as above.
- *Concurrent validity*. This applies when the researcher employs a test on groups known to differ and in a way relevant to the concept under study.
- *Predictive validity*. This applies where a test is applied and the subject group is followed up to determine whether the test can predict those subjects who will develop some condition.
- *Convergent validity*. This is a more general term. It includes the above measures of validity and refers to the process whereby the measure is tested for harmonization with some pre-existing measure. However, Bryman & Cramer note that using different methods is more useful than the more common application of convergent validity testing where similar methods (e.g. two questionnaires) are employed.
- *Divergent validity*. The idea here is that measures of different concepts should not correspond with each other; in other words, the measures discriminate.

All the above descriptions of validity are open to some question, but it is nonetheless useful to consider them. For example, it is possible for a group of experts to be wrong about the relevance of an item (content validity), as there may be systematic errors in the field. Consider the field of medicine, where a normal pineal or adrenal gland was taken to be a symptom of disease (due to the practise of doing post-mortems on the poor, who had enlarged adrenal and pineal glands). Construct validity is not necessarily disproven by doctoral students being shown to be of similar intellect to students unable to gain entry to university; perhaps the doctoral students were from a privileged background rather than inherently more intelligent. A new highly superior measuring device may not show much similarity with an inferior older device; furthermore, perhaps the older device was itself not valid. However, the least that can be said if experts consider your questionnaire items irrelevant or badly formed, or if a pilot sample cannot understand your questionnaire, or if there is no difference found between two groups where you expect a difference, or if your instrument is not even similar to a well tried and trusted device, is that you should seriously consider the validity of your instrument (be it a questionnaire, a physical measurement device or an interview question).

RELIABILITY

If a measure is *repeatable* then we should get the same result when we measure the same thing twice (or more). Reliability measures give a quantitative value for repeatability. For example, they may be used to assess how repeatable a machine is, or to what extent two humans give the same value.

Stability: test–retest

This tests whether a measuring device (which could be a human) gives the same result when the measurement is repeated. Typically, the measurements could be physical measurements, and the correlation between one score and the other is calculated. A high correlation is a necessary, but not sufficient, condition for stability. For example, a high correlation could be obtained if the second measure were exactly half that of the first occasion. There are problems with this technique, especially where the testing of humans using, say, some form of skills test. In such a case if too little time is left between measurements the subject may have remembered enough to change the re-test score, but if a large time lag is allowed it could be argued that any changes noted are real (i.e. not an artefact or error).

Equivalence: comparing two forms of test or two observers

If two observers are involved in a study (inter-rater reliability), then we would want them to give the same score. However, in practice there will always be some discrepancies. For example, two lecturers will almost always give different marks to the same piece of work, although there may still be an overall trend to agreement.

One way of assessing equivalence is to calculate

Number of agreements
Number of possible agreements

Suppose two student nurses assess a group of patients for grade of sore, where the sore could be described as superficial or deep. To simplify the example let us assume that there are the same number of patients with superficial as with deep sores (as assessed by an expert in tissue viability). If the nurses agreed on the type of sore all the time their assessment would be said to be reliable, but in practice they will sometimes disagree. Suppose they agreed half of the time, then one would say that the assessment was 50% reliable. But in fact there are only two possibilities (superficial or deep sore), and so if the two nurses were guessing all the time you would expect them to agree at about this level.

Now suppose that the sores were graded on a scale of 1–4, where 1 indicates a reddened area and 4 indicates a deep cavity sore, with scores of 2 and 3 indicating intermediate sores. Assume there are equal numbers of sores of each level. If the two nurses agreed about half the time on the grading of the sores they are in fact doing rather well, for by chance they would agree only about 25% of the time (one time in four).

So the number of possible classifications is important – clearly it is easier to guess correctly a yes/no answer than an answer to a multiple choice question with four possible answers (this is entirely analogous to the two examples given for sore assessment).

Example: X-ray diagnosis

Interpretation of medical images is an area where two humans will not always agree, even if they are experienced. However, you would ordinarily assume that a very experienced observer, such as a consultant radiologist, would give the correct interpretation of straightforward radiographs of possible fractures. For example, Overton[3] compared the diagnoses of distal fractures as made by a consultant radiologist and by several nurses and doctors. Here, however, we will concentrate on just one nurse and compare her with the radiologist.

In this example 18 cases were diagnosed as fracture by both the radiologist and the nurse, 24 were diagnosed as normal by both the radiologist and the nurse, and there were 5 cases where the nurse thought there was a fracture and the radiologist considered it normal, and 3 cases where the radiologist thought there was a fracture and the nurse considered it normal, making 50 cases in total.

An apparently reasonable measure of agreement is to work out the ratio of those radiographs that the nurse and radiologist agree on:

$$\text{Agreement} = \frac{18 + 24}{50}$$
$$= 0.82 \text{ (or 82\%)}$$

However, to see why this is not necessarily a good idea, consider the (fictional) case where there were only a few cases (say 5 out of 50) diagnosed as fractures by the radiologist, and further suppose that the nurse had no idea which radiographs were abnormal and guessed all the time. To make things worse, let us suppose that the nurse always got it wrong (fairly unlikely), and allocated 90% (45) images to the normal group. We would then have 5 cases where there was in fact a fracture that the nurse missed, and 5 normals that she identified as a fracture, but she would still agree with the radiologist on the 40 other images, giving an agreement of 0.80 or 80%, much as above. So, not only is the possible number of classifications important, but the frequency of occurrence of each possible answer matters. Here we have only two possible outcomes, fracture or normal, but it is *not* the case that a random agreement will be 50%. As we have seen above, by knowing the overall frequencies you can guess much more effectively than this. An analogous situation would be if you were completing a multiple choice exam and were told that most (say three-quarters) of the correct answers were the third of four items, by always stating the answer to be number three you would get 75% of the questions right even if you did not know the correct answer to any question.

If the nurse had allocated five patients at random to the fracture group, she would probably do a little better. The (random) classification rate can be calculated from the contingency table (see Ch. 5) of the diagnoses made by the two professionals. The fictional case is given in Table 3.1. A nurse guessing would be allocating according to the probabilities given by the marginal totals, i.e.

$$P_c = \frac{1}{N} \sum \frac{n_{i.} \, n_{.i}}{N}$$

where N is the total number of cases, $n_{i.}$ is the ith row total and $n_{.i}$ the ith column total, so the agreement found by chance would be:

$$P_c = \frac{1}{50} \left(\frac{45 \times 45}{50} + \frac{5 \times 5}{50} \right) = \frac{1}{50} (40.5 + 0.5) = 0.82$$

So we get the same value for the (fictional) random diagnosis as for the agreement found in (real) practice. Does this mean the agreement of 0.82 found by Overton[3] does not indicate any real diagnostic skill by the nurse?

The answer is not necessarily, it depends on the relative numbers of fractures versus normals, in the real case the contingency table is as shown in Table 3.2. We have

Table 3.1

Nurse	Radiologist		
	Normal	Fracture	Total
Normal	40	5	45
Fracture	5	0	5
Total	45	5	50

Table 3.2

Nurse	Radiologist		
	Normal	Fracture	Total
Normal	24	5	29
Fracture	3	18	21
Total	27	23	50

$$P_c = \frac{1}{50}\left(\frac{29 \times 27}{50} + \frac{21 \times 23}{50}\right) = \frac{1}{50}(15.67 + 9.66) = 0.51$$

So in this case we would expect an agreement of about one-half (51%) of the time by *chance alone*; however, the value of 0.82 is in excess of this.

A more meaningful measure of association that takes into account the possibility of getting random agreement is kappa (κ).[4] This measure has many attractive features:

- Complete agreement is given by a value of 1.0
- Agreement due to chance (i.e. random) gives a value of 0.0
- It may be used on nominal measures.

A good description of kappa is given in Professor Everitt's excellent monograph,[5] which is referred to in the chapter on contingency tables (Ch. 5). Kappa is defined as:

$$\kappa = \frac{P_o - P_c}{1 - P_c}$$

where P_o is the value observed. In the cases above, since $P_o = P_c$ for the random (fictional) case, then $\kappa = 0$, and for the actual values found by Overton[3]

$$\kappa = \frac{0.82 - 0.51}{0.49} = 0.63$$

Everitt[5] describes strengths of agreement (attributed to Landis & Koch[6]) indicated by the value of κ:

0.0–0.20   Poor agreement
0.21–0.40   Fair agreement
0.41–0.60   Moderate agreement
0.61–0.80   Substantial agreement
0.81–1.00   Almost perfect agreement

So, on the above scale, the agreement between the nurse and the consultant radiologist is substantial.

The above two cases should give no cause for surprise. As, in the real case, about half of the radiographs were normal, if the nurse guessed then a value of 50% is what you would expect. The fictional case where the number of fractures is very small as a percentage is understandable, as the nurse may know the rough ratio of fractures in her clinic (about 10%) and so allocate one in 10 to a fracture. Although she does not really know which of the radiographs show fractures, she is still able to score a high agreement with the specialist, as most radiographs are normal and she allocates most to a normal group.

Table 3.3

Observer 1	Observer 2	Agree
1	1	Yes
1	1	Yes
0	0	Yes
0	0	Yes
1	1	Yes
0	0	Yes
1	0	No
1	1	Yes
1	1	Yes
1	1	Yes
1	1	Yes
1	1	Yes
1	1	Yes
1	1	Yes
1	1	Yes
1	1	Yes
0	1	No
1	0	No
1	0	No
1	1	Yes

0, Scintigram normal; 1, Scintigram abnormal.

Table 3.4

Physicist 2	Physicist 1 Normal	Abnormal	Total
Normal	3	1	4
Abnormal	3	13	16
Total	6	14	20

In another study two medical physicists were compared to see if they agreed with each other in their analysis of nuclear scintigrams.[7] The scintigrams were diagnosed either as normal or as abnormal, as shown in Table 3.3 (where zero means normal, and one means abnormality). A cross-tabulation of these data is given in Table 3.4. We have

$$P_c = \frac{1}{20}\left(\frac{4 \times 6}{20} + \frac{16 \times 14}{20}\right) = \frac{1}{20}\left(\frac{24}{20} + \frac{224}{20}\right) = 0.62$$

In fact they agreed in 16 out of 20 cases, so $P_o = 0.80$, and

$$\kappa = \frac{P_o - P_c}{1 - P_c} = \frac{0.80 - 0.62}{1 - 0.62} = 0.47$$

so this apparently similar result (80% agreement) is by the criterion of kappa only a moderate agreement.

SPSS allows you to perform a kappa analysis via the *Statistics* pull-down, by clicking on Summarize and then Crosstabs, and you select the two variables, one as a row and the other as a column (i.e. as if you were doing a chi square (χ^2) analysis). In this case the data are the values given by each observer for each case. The data are paired: each row is for one case, and the two variables are the values assigned by the two observers.

The Output screen for the medical imaging example shown in Figure 3.1. The variables OB1 and OB2 contain the values ascribed by the two observers. Note that the value given is the same as the one we found by direct calculation. Furthermore, a significance level is given, which at $p = 0.028$ is below our usual α level (< 0.05), so we may be quite confident that the agreement did not occur by chance.

Intra-class correlation coefficient

If continuous (at least ordinal) data are used, then the correlation coefficient can be employed to give a value of repeatability. A repeated measures correlation coefficient is often called the *reliability* of the measurement method.[8] However there are problems in using this method. As noted above, a repeated measure could be double the value of the first measure, and yet give a correlation of unity. If the order of the values is important (and using a correlation technique implicitly makes the

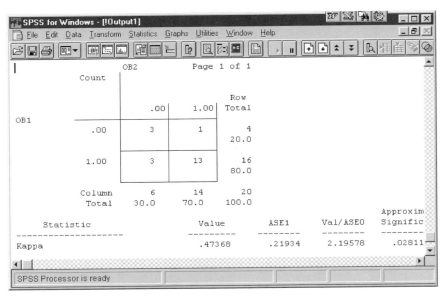

Figure 3.1   Kappa analysis: SPSS Output screen.

assumption that this is not the case), then reversing the order of some of the paired values will alter the coefficient.

In such a case a better measure is the intra-class correlation coefficient, which estimates the average correlation among all possible pairs of observations. Unfortunately, a means of calculating this coefficient is not available in most computer packages. However, if the number of observations is the same for each subject we can use the following equation:[8]

$$r_i = \frac{mSS_B - SS_T}{(m-1)SS_T}$$

where r_i is the intra-class correlation coefficient, m is the number of observations, SS_T is the total sum of squares and SS_B is the between-subjects sum of squares (also called within-groups sum of squares). SS_B and SS_T can be obtained via a one-way ANOVA (see Ch. 6).

In the above example of scintigrams assessed by medical physicists, the images were in fact given a range of values from -4 to $+4$, and not merely normal or abnormal. One way ANOVA gave the output shown in Figure 3.2. Here $m = 2$, and r_i is given by

$$r_i = \frac{2 \times 186.85 - 188.975}{1 \times 188.975}$$

$$= 0.98 \text{ (to two decimal places)}$$

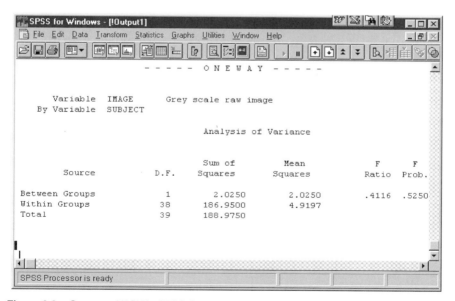

Figure 3.2   One way ANOVA: SPSS Output screen.

However, given the limited number of possible values that could be returned, this very high correlation is not as impressive as it appears.

INTERNAL RELIABILITY

The validity measures described above are examples of *external* reliability. However, in a questionnaire, for example, you might want to see if the items within the questionnaire are measuring the same thing, i.e. whether they show *internal* reliability.

If you want to measure an attitude, for example, then you might have a questionnaire with several questions that aim to address this particular aspect. The reason for asking more than one question would typically be to gain a more accurate measure by averaging responses over several items, thus reducing the possibility of single idiosyncratic responses unduly affecting the measure. This is similar in concept to asking many questions in an examination (say a multiple choice examination), where all the questions concern the same subject; an average of these forms a better basis for assessment than asking one question.

You would want the questions in the attitude (or knowledge) question-naire to show some correlation with each other, for if they did not then they are probably not measuring the same thing. A new questionnaire should be checked for internal reliability, or homogeneity. Various methods exist, of which the most common are split-half and Cronbach's α. In either case a value close to zero indicates that the questions are not addressing the same item, and a value near 1 means that they are. Values over about 0.7–0.8 are generally considered adequate. If you obtain very low values for internal reliability then you should probably remove some items.

Note: You might consider that what is described here as internal reliability is really internal validity, as we are exploring the relevance of items to be included in a cluster of items that are to measure some construct. I have some sympathy with this view, and in some texts you may see the measures described below classified as measures of validity. However, I am following the terminology used in both SPSS and several texts (e.g. Bryman & Cramer[9]).

Split-half technique

In the split-half technique the items are split into two groups, and these two groups are correlated with each other. In SPSS you select Statistics, then Scale, then Reliability Analysis. This gives the dialogue box shown in Figure 3.3. Here a questionnaire composed of two constructs has been used. The items are distributed throughout the questionnaire, such that questions 1, 4, 5, 6, 10, 11 and 14 are designed to form one construct, and the remaining questions (2, 3, 7, 8, 9, 12, 13 and 15) correspond to the other

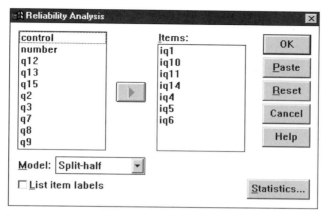

Figure 3.3   Split-half reliability analysis: SPSS dialogue box.

construct. The variables iq1, iq4, iq5, iq6, iq10, iq11 and iq14 correspond to the questions in the first set, and have been entered into the analysis.

In split-half tests the first half of the variables are correlated with the second half, and thus the technique is sensitive to the order in which the variables are entered. As can be seen in Figure 3.4, the questionnaire shows a fair internal validity. The correlation between the two sets of variables is given as 0.41 (to two decimal places) and overall reliability 0.51.

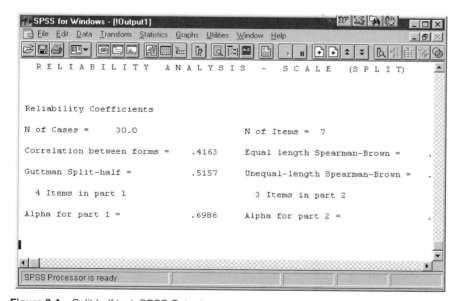

Figure 3.4   Split-half test: SPSS Output screen.

Cronbach α

In the split-half test the order in which the variables are entered into the analysis affects the result. Cronbach's α, however, considers all the correlations among all the variables and reports the average of these. Thus it is not sensitive to the ordering of variables, and may be considered a more robust measure. it is a very commonly seen test for internal reliability in the literature, and is the default in SPSS (Fig. 3.5).

A coefficient of 1.0 indicates perfect agreement among the items (i.e. they all measure exactly the same thing) and logically, therefore, all but one could be removed from the instrument. An α coefficient of zero indicates no agreement at all among the items. Thus the items are not measuring the same thing, and are therefore not useful if being used as a battery of variables to measure some attribute. A high coefficient (typically above 0.7) shows that the variables are probably measuring the same thing, and are plausible for use as a cluster of variables to measure an attribute.

Note that these measures of internal reliability do not prove or disprove that collections of variables are useful measures of an attribute. It would be possible to use a set of variables that are internally reliable but measure something completely different to what you wanted to measure. A set of questions meant to measure depression could, for example, be measuring anxiety. However, as a check on your (typically survey) instrument

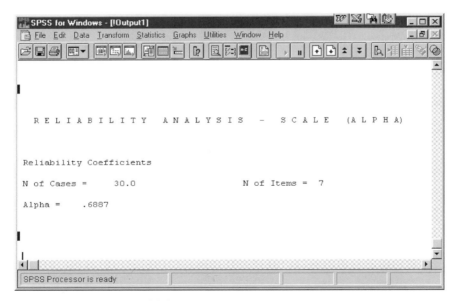

Figure 3.5 Cronbach α: SPSS Output screen.

internal reliability measures should alert you to the plausibility of the items.

In the case illustrated here, the Cronbach α of 0.69 (to two places of decimals) indicates a moderately high internal validity.

CONCLUSION

Validity and reliability are measures of the quality of your study. Validity assesses the relevance of the items in your research tool, i.e. whether they measure what they are supposed to measure. External reliability assesses how well the instrument performs when measures are repeated, either over time or by different observers. Internal reliability is concerned with the correct clustering of items designed to measure the same construct.

EXERCISES

1. The Waterlow score gives an indication of the risk of developing pressure sores. It is based on 11 components (e.g. continence and mobility), all of which are measured on a numerical scale. Using the criterion that all patients with a Waterlow score over 10 are at danger of developing sores, the prediction of sore development (PRED; 0 = no sore will develop, or 1 = a sore will develop) was compared with the actual outcome (SORE; 0 = no sore developed, 1 = a sore developed). The following output was given by SPSS for Cohen's κ. Interpret the result, and comment on the strength and significance of the κ value.

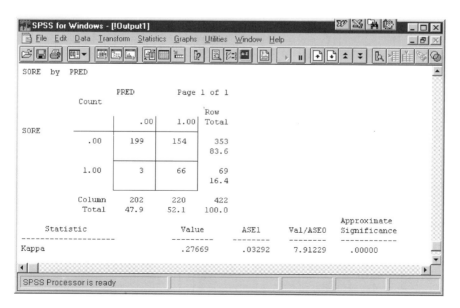

2. The 11 components of the Waterlow score were analysed using the α test. The output from SPSS is shown below. Comment on the result. Do you think the components are measuring the same thing?

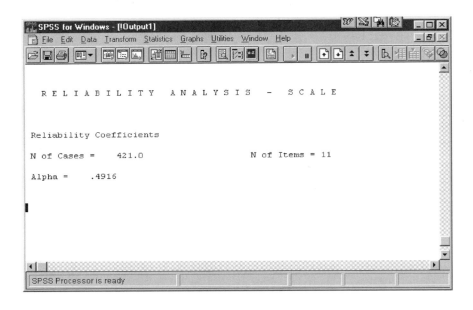

REFERENCES

1. Dempsey P A, Dempsey A D 1996 Nursing research: Text and workbook. Little, Brown, Boston, M A, p 69–70
2. Bryman A, Cramer D 1997 Quantitative data analysis. Routledge, London, p 65–67
3. Overton P 1996 Towards a partnership in care: Nurses' and doctors' interpretation of extremity trauma radiology. Masters Thesis, University of Birmingham, UK
4. Cohen J 1960 A coefficient of agreement for nominal scales. Educational and Psychological Measurement 20: 37–46
5. Everitt B S 1992 The analysis of contingency tables. Chapman & Hall, London, p 146–150
6. Landis J R, Koch G G 1977 The measurement of observer agreement for categorical data. Biometrics 33: 117–129
7. Anthony D M 1988 An exploration in the use of pre-processes and colour displays in nuclear medicine images. Masters Thesis, University of Warwick, UK
8. Bland J M, Altman D G 1996 Measurement error and correlation coefficients. British Medical Journal 313: 41–42
9. Bryman A, Cramer D 1997 Quantitative data analysis. Routledge, London, p 62–67

4

Correlation and partial correlation

Simple correlation is a topic covered well in most texts. It is so crucial to other chapters of this book, for example correlation is the basis for other more powerful techniques such as regression, factor analysis (FA) and principal components analysis (PCA), that it is discussed here in some detail. However, for an introduction you could look at almost any basic statistics text. One text specific to SPSS is that by Bryman & Cramer[1] and you could also look at the SPSS manual.[2]

KEY POINTS

- Correlation assumes linearity

- Correlation does not prove causality

- Significance of a correlation coefficient is required before interpretation can be made

- Partial correlation techniques can help to suggest possible causative relationships

- Partial correlation can suggest, though not prove, possible artefacts in apparent relationships

At the end of this chapter the student should be able to:

1. State an appropriate correlation test given a data distribution

2. Interpret a correlation coefficient

3. Identify the four relationships that partial correlation may help uncover

4. Interpret a partial correlation coefficient

SIMPLE CORRELATION

The basic idea behind correlation is that two variables are related to each other in a linear fashion. *Linear* means that the relationship is modelled as a straight line. Figure 4.1 shows such a relationship, where as one variable x increases, so does y. In this case y is exactly twice x at each point, and the relationship is described as $y = 2x$, and when $x = 0$ so also $y = 0$, i.e. the line goes through the origin of the graph. In general, however, it is possible for one variable to be non-zero when the other equals zero, i.e. the line does not go through the origin. The more general formula for a straight line would be $y = mx + c$, where y is one variable, x is the other variable, and m and c are constants. The equation $y = 2x$ is thus a special case where $c = 0$ and $m = 2$. With a clear and straightforward relationship like this, you can see that if you know the value of one variable you can predict exactly what the value of the other variable will be. Specifically, if $x = 3$ then $y = 6$, etc.

However, such simple relationships are rare in the natural world. A

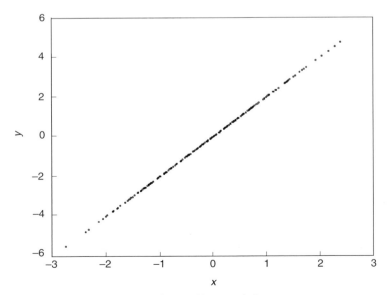

Figure 4.1   A linear relationship: perfect positive correlation.

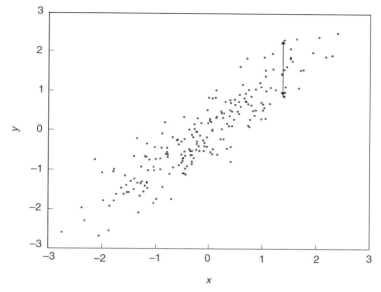

Figure 4.2   A positive correlation less than unity.

more typical relationship is shown in Figure 4.2, where a scatterplot (this is what SPSS calls such a figure, but it is variously referred to as a scattergraph, scattergram or scatter diagram) shows that a similar relationship exists as the one in Figure 4.1. As one variable increases so does the other. However, one variable cannot be predicted exactly from the other. In this case while in general as x increases, y increases, you cannot be absolutely sure what one variable will be, given the other. If you look at any particular value of x you will note that there may be several possible points, each with a different y value. Consider the vertical line: it has four points on or very near to it that range in their y value from about 1 to more than 2. Yet the relationship, while inexact, is still very obvious.

In SPSS a scatterplot is obtained via the Graphs pull-down menu. In the simplest case, you would select two variables, which are plotted against each other so that each point on the diagram is created from the two values for the variables – you look across to the y axis and down to the x axis from each point to see the values of the two variables.

Yet another relationship is shown in Figure 4.3, where one variable decreases as the other increases. This shows a similar degree of relationship, but in the opposite direction.

These three cases are examples of correlation. The first (Fig. 4.1) shows a *perfect correlation*, and this is given a value of unity, or 1.0. This is the

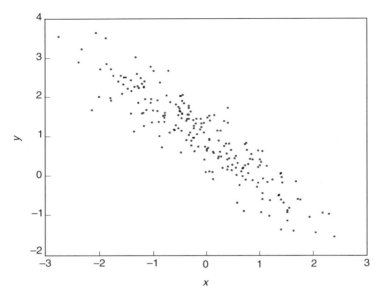

Figure 4.3   A negative correlation less than unity.

highest correlation possible. If the two variables are not related in any way (i.e. there is no correlation), then the correlation is zero, which is the lowest correlation. The plot in Figure 4.2 is somewhere in between. The correlation is not perfect, but a relationship clearly exists. The correlation will be somewhere between zero and 1.0. Any correlation that is greater than zero is said to be a positive correlation. Finally, a negative relationship, or *negative correlation* (Fig. 4.3), is lower than zero. But the negative correlation is not less than a zero correlation; the negative sign indicates the direction of the relationship, and the absolute value indicates the amount of correlation. Thus a correlation of − 0.5 and a correlation of + 0.5 show the same amount of correlation, but in different directions.

Correlation is only meaningful if the underlying relationship is linear, or can at least be modelled as linear (in some cases a non-linear relationship may be linear within a given range, or may be converted to a linear relation by some transformation, typically by taking logarithms). Thus in some cases, for example the plot shown in Figure 4.4, a correlation of zero would be found; despite an obvious relationship, correlation is not an appropriate measure. Figure 4.4 is a quadratic relationship, not linear.

A correlation coefficient can be between − 1 and + 1. The higher the absolute value (i.e. the value where the negative sign is removed) the higher the correlation, and the sign indicates the direction of the relationship.

SPSS gives correlation coefficients for normal (parametric) and non-

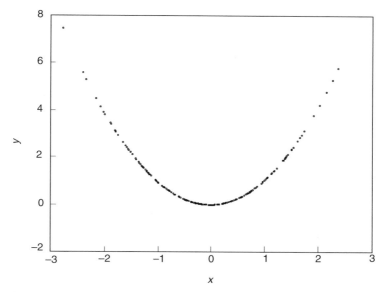

Figure 4.4   A non-linear (quadratic in this case) relationship.

normal distributions. They are both obtainable via the Statistics pull-down, by clicking on Correlate and then Bivariate. The two variables are given in the resulting dialogue box, and you can choose Pearson, Spearman or Kendal's tau (τ). The Pearson test assumes a normal distribution, and is a parametric test; the other two are non-parametric tests and perform similarly, although the Spearman test is more commonly used. Kendal's τ typically gives a slightly smaller coefficient, but otherwise there is little to choose between the two tests.

All three tests have the same interpretation, they all return a correlation coefficient and a p value. A lot of confusion reigns between the two values. While for most statistical tests only the p value need be reported, in correlation the actual coefficient is important. However, the coefficient is only meaningful if the p value is lower than the α level used (typically 0.05). Thus we can have several different scenarios:

- *A* p *value higher than the* α *level.* In this case the size and direction of the correlation coefficient is meaningless, whatever its size.
- *A* p *value lower than the* α *level.* In this case the correlation coefficient is worth considering, and may be any value (except zero) between −1 and + 1, depending on the size of the sample.
- In particular, there are four possible cases: a high or low correlation that is significant; or a high or low correlation that is not significant. You should not confuse the p value with the degree of correlation.

Sample size affects the correlation coefficient that can be found to be significant. A very small sample will only allow a large (absolute) coefficient to exceed statistical significance. Larger samples will allow smaller coefficients to reach significance. In extreme cases you may find significant correlation coefficients that are tiny, and of no real *clinical* significance. This is similar to when a large sample shows a tiny but significant difference between two group means when Student's *t*-test is used.

Pearson and Spearman rank tests

An example of using correlation is given in Figure 4.5, which shows the relationship between the results obtained by students in the research examination and the research dissertation of a nursing course

The data show a Pearson correlation. You may elect to perform the correlation coefficient between more than two variables (in which case several correlations will be computed on a pairwise basis, so for variables *A*, *B* and *C* the correlations for *A* versus *B*, *B* versus *C*, and *A* versus *C* would be computed), in which case SPSS would show this as a display similar to the mileage charts in some atlases, showing the distance between towns. In the example shown in Figure 4.5 there are only two variables, but SPSS still shows all possible correlations: RESEAR3 versus RESEAR4,

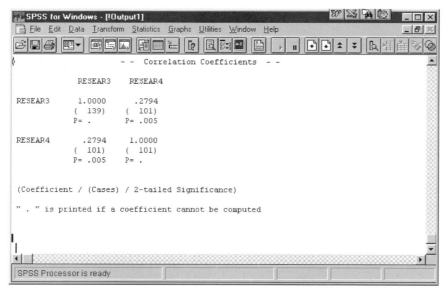

Figure 4.5 Pearson correlation of two variables: SPSS Output screen.

but also RESEAR4 versus RESEAR3, which is the same; and the other trivial correlations RESEAR3 versus RESEAR3, and RESEAR4 versus RESEAR4. Thus we get the unsurprising result that RESEAR3 is perfectly correlated with itself, as is RESEAR4 (in both cases SPSS records the p value as a decimal point, indicating it cannot work out a correlation coefficient that is meaningful). In each case the probability cannot be computed (the relationship is trivial and not interesting anyway). The other two correlations are the same, and this is also unsurprising. The correlation coefficient is not dependent on the order of the two variables, any more than the distance between London and Glasgow is any different than that between Glasgow and London. Thus the above box boils down to a Pearson's correlation of 0.2794 with a p value of 0.005. The interpretation is that a small positive correlation exists between the examination and the dissertation results and that this correlation is highly significant.

Suppose we were to discover that the data were non-normal. In this case we could choose the Spearman test, and would get the results shown in Figure 4.6. In this case SPSS reaches the sensible conclusion that there are only two variables, and thus there is only any point in giving *one* correlation coefficient. In fact, if you elect to have more than two variables you get only the lower triangle of the whole matrix, unlike the Pearson test where a square array is reported (see below for examples of how SPSS reports three variables). The correlation of RESEAR3 with RESEAR4 in

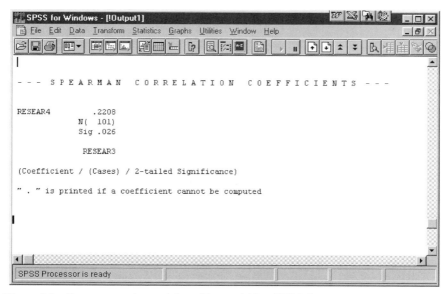

Figure 4.6 Spearman rank correlation of two variables: SPSS Output screen.

this case gives a very similar result, i.e. a small positive correlation that is highly significant. In general this may not be the case, and you should report the result of the test that is most appropriate, given the nature of the distribution.

Now consider the case of three variables (Figs 4.7 and 4.8). We can see that BRANCH3, which is a branch-specific module (the course consists of three branches, for child health nursing, adult nursing and mental health nursing; in the final two years of the degree students undertake some common modules, but split into three branches for specialist modules relating to their chosen branch), shows a small significant negative correlation with RESEAR4, and a smaller and non-significant one with RESEAR3, using either the Spearman or the Pearson test. Other differences in the reporting are that for Pearson's correlation the heading of the Output screen does not tell you which test is being used, although in the case of Spearman's test it does tell you which version is being used for correlation. Furthermore, for the Spearman test the significance is denoted by Sig, and for Pearson it is denoted by P=.

You might wonder why SPSS does not report the correlation coefficients in a consistent manner. The answer almost certainly lies in the use of different programmers to write the two procedures, with no editing done by SPSS to improve the look and feel of the product. This seems to be a typical feature of SPSS, where each component (even within the same pull-down menu) shows items such as the *p* value in a different fashion.

```
        - - Correlation Coefficients - -

            RESEAR3    RESEAR4    BRANCH3

RESEAR3     1.0000      .2794     -.0414
          (  139)     (  101)    (  101)
          P= .        P= .005    P= .681

RESEAR4      .2794     1.0000      .2634
          (  101)     (  101)    (  101)
          P= .005     P= .       P= .008

BRANCH3     -.0414      .2634     1.0000
          (  101)     (  101)    (  101)
          P= .681     P= .008    P= .

(Coefficient / (Cases) / 2-tailed Significance)

" . " is printed if a coefficient cannot be computed
```

Figure 4.7 Pearson pairwise correlation of three variables: SPSS Output screen.

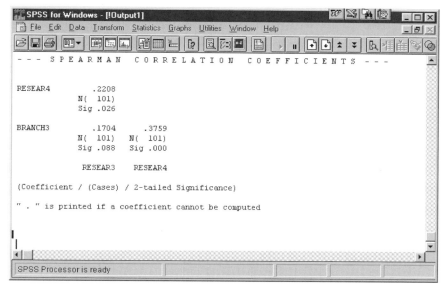

Figure 4.8   Spearman rank pairwise correlation of three variables: SPSS Output screen.

This I find a little odd (and irritating), as SPSS is a very mature product, having been around for many years.

As an example of where the correlation test is useful, consider Figure 4.9. There is no obvious correlation between x and y. I could persuade myself that a small tendency to increase y with increasing x may be present; however, I could also be easily persuaded that the points are simply random. A Pearson's test (the data are normally distributed) gives a correlation coefficient $r = 0.29$ and $p < 0.001$. Thus although the correlation coefficient is low, the relationship is highly significant, and this can be seen only when a test is applied.

The size of the correlation coefficient needs to be interpreted with care. As seen in the chapter on power analysis (Ch. 12), a correlation coefficient of $r = 0.1$ means that 1% of the variance of one variable is apparently explained by the other, but a higher value of $r = 0.5$ means that 25% of the variance of one variable is apparently explained by the other. Thus a correlation five times as large explains 25 times the variance. To give a better description of the size of the correlation the squared correlation coefficient r^2 is often used, and this is called the *coefficient of determination*. This value gives the exact amount of variance accounted for by the correlation coefficient; thus $r = 0.1$ gives $r^2 = 0.01$, and $r = 0.5$ gives $r^2 = 0.25$, or 1% and 25%, respectively. As a further example $r = 1.0$ gives $r^2 = 1$ (100%), as expected; this is twice the value of a correlation coefficient of $r = 0.5$, but explains four times the variance.

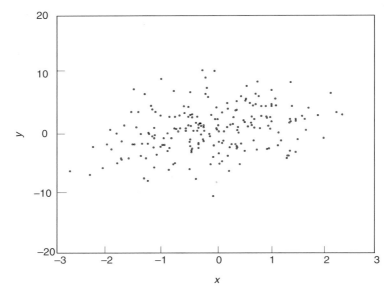

Figure 4.9 A plot of data showing little or no correlation.

Conditions of correlation

We have already stated that correlation assumes linearity, but there are other considerations to take into account. The main conditions are:

- *Linearity.* Only linear relations are appropriate for correlation.
- *Extrapolation.* While you may interpolate within data that appear correlated, extrapolating beyond the range of data upon which the correlation has been computed is not permitted. It may be the case that two variables may be correlated within a range of values, but not outside of those values. For example, in Figure 4.4 the relationship is roughly linear from $x = -3$ to $x = -1$, and a negative correlation between x and y would be a fair model. However, the curve then makes a sharp bend around $x = 0$, and then from $x = 1$ to $x = 3$ you could describe it as roughly linear again, but this time as a positive correlation. Therefore, if all you had was the scatterplot for the values between $x = -3$ to $x = -1$ then your prediction for the rest of the values of y given x would be totally wrong. An example might be the effect of a drug on the body, say alcohol. Initially, increasing intake makes you feel better, a positive correlation of dose and feeling of well-being; however, this relationship does not last, as very large doses of alcohol make you feel worse, not better.
- *Variance.* If the variances of the two variables are very different, the correlation coefficient will be smaller than if both the variables had a similar variance.

- *Homoscedasticity.* The points about a regression line (see Ch. 7) should show no pattern, in the sense that the range of data is the same at each point of the line.
- *Outliers:* A few, or even one, very extreme values can affect the correlation coefficient. This is only a problem with the parametric test.

To test for linearity you should first construct a scatterplot, which will show major departures from linearity. Homoscedasticity should be clear by inspecting the range of y values for each value of x. If the ranges are very different then the opposite of heteroscedasticity would be observed. For example, in Figure 4.2 the range of values of y for each value of x is similar. The effect of range is also immediately seen in a graph. For example, in Figure 4.2 it would be unwise to assume that correlation continued to be valid outside the values of y in the range $[-3, +3]$, as it is within this range of values that the coefficient has been computed.

You should also be very cautious about making assumptions of causality; the fact that two variables are correlated does not mean one causes the other. Furthermore, even if such a relation does hold, the correlation coefficient gives no indication of which is the cause and which is the effect. For example, if poverty were shown to be correlated with ill health (as it in fact is), then it is not clear whether ill health causes you to become poor (e.g. through reduced income because of unemployment caused through ill health), or whether after becoming unemployed, say, and thus being on a lower income, health deteriorates. While it is generally assumed that the cause is poverty and the effect ill health, the evidence is not directly obtainable via a correlation coefficient, but rather from more detailed observations such as time series, where workers are monitored before and after unemployment, and compared with matched samples.

Nominal data correlation measures

There are also measures of correlation that may be applied to nominal data. The chi square (χ^2) test measures the independence of two variables, but in SPSS you can elect in the χ^2 dialogue box (see Ch. 5) to be given the phi (ϕ; recommended for 2×2 tables) or Cramer's V (recommended for larger tables) test result. Cramer's V gives coefficients that range between zero and 1, the values having a similar interpretation as the other correlation coefficients mentioned above. The concept of negative correlation exists for nominal data only in the case of the ϕ value, which ranges between -1 and $+1$ in the same way as in the Pearson and Spearman rank tests. (*Note:* As Bryman & Cramer[3] note, in some texts Cramer's V takes on both positive and negative values. This is not the case when using the formula adopted in SPSS, which is a particular variant that allows only positive values.)

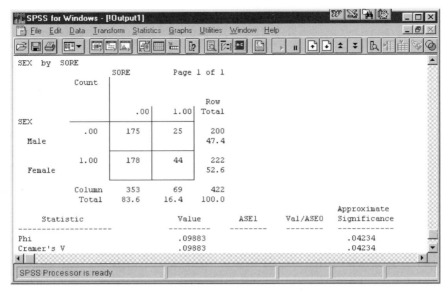

Figure 4.10 Values of φ and Cramer's *V*: SPSS Output screen.

The φ and Cramer's *V* tests check association rather than independence, and give a numerical value that indicates the strength of the association.

In the Waterlow score data (see Ch. 3), gender was thought to be associated with sore formation. The scores recorded for hospital patients are given in Figure 4.10. Note the absolute value of the result, and the significance of the φ and Cramer's *V* values are identical. This will always be the case for a 2×2 table, but not in general. The results show a small but significant (positive) correlation between gender and sores. In this case, as can be seen for the expected values (given under the actual observed values), male patients had fewer sores than expected, and female patients more than expected, and the direction of the φ value (positive) indicates increasing value for gender from 0 (male) to 1 (female) increases sores from 0 (no sore) to 1 (sore), which says the same thing. The Waterlow score does in fact give a higher score to females than to males, which these results indicate is appropriate, although work on wheelchair users (e.g.) casts doubt on this being a general rule.[4,5]

PARTIAL CORRELATION

Partial correlation is explained in the SPSS manual[6] and discussed in Bryman & Cramer.[7] The assumption behind partial correlation is that a variable may be correlated with more than one other variable, and that a simple relationship between two variables is not realistic in such cases.

In particular, partial correlation is designed to uncover four types of relationship:

- *Spurious correlations.* In this case a correlation may be seen between two variables that may be large and highly relevant. Closer examination reveals that both variables are related to a third variable, and the two variables have no real relationship. For example, if the number of newspapers read were correlated with air quality there may be (this is imaginary) a correlation of 0.6. However reading newspapers is unlikely to reduce air quality. What may be the case is that increased emission of toxic gases from industrial plants is an effect of industrialization, and another effect of industrialization is rising literacy, which is needed for the more educated workforce required in this more technological age.
- *Intervening variables.* In this case one variable effects a second variable, which itself effects a third variable. That is, one variable is a product of the independent variable and a cause of the dependent variable.[8]
- *Moderated relationships.* In this case a relationship holds for some categories of a variable, but not all.
- *Multiple causation.* This is where more than one independent variable is the cause of the dependent variable.

It is not possible to use partial correlation to test for the presence of each of the above relationships in the absence of any other information. However, it can help identify likely relationships given prior knowledge.

For Waterlow scores a correlation of 0.4666 ($p < 0.001$) was found between the skin subscore and age. However, perhaps skin is adversely affected by mobility rather than age, and the pertinent fact is that older people tend to be more restricted in mobility. Allowing for mobility gives a correlation of 0.3807 and $p < 0.001$ (Fig. 4.11). It is clear that allowing for mobility reduces the correlation, but in which particular way could this be? Let us consider the following possibilities:

- Spurious correlations. If the apparent relationship between age and skin were in fact due to mobility alone, which itself is related to age, then the apparent relationship would disappear when mobility was allowed for. This did not happen, so if the relationship is spurious, then mobility is not the root cause. There is no evidence of a spurious relationship (although this could still could be so, but not explicable by the mobility variable).
- Intervening variables. For a similar reason the results would not be explicable by an intervening variable of mobility. The theory would now be that age causes loss of mobility, and it is this loss of mobility that actually causes the sore. However, again the correlation would be reduced to zero once mobility was allowed for, and this did not happen. Incidentally, knowledge of the domain allows us to reject the possibility of an

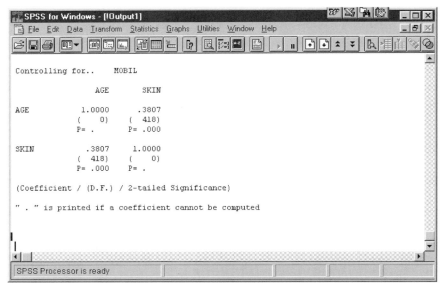

Figure 4.11 Partial correlation coefficients: SPSS Output screen.

intervening variable in the other direction – as it is clearly implausible that loss of mobility causes us to grow older, and that age is an intervening variable in the mobility and skin subscores.

• Moderated relationship. The best way to test for moderated relationships is to perform a correlation test on more than one category of the proposed moderator.[9] For example, a correlation test could be done on skin versus age for low mobility and on skin versus age for high mobility. In this case an $r = 0.2388$ ($p = 0.003$) was found for a mobility of 0, $r = 0.3567$ for a mobility of 3, and $r = 0.4617$ for a mobility of 4 (all other values of mobility were non-significant). Thus there does appear to be some evidence that mobility moderates for the relationship between skin and age, in the sense that the relationship becomes more pronounced as the mobility value increases (i.e. as mobility gets less).

• Multiple causation. As allowing for mobility does not remove the effect of age on skin, mobility cannot be the sole cause of skin deterioration. We might imagine that mobility has little impact on skin; however, a partial correlation of skin with mobility allowing for age gives a moderate and highly significant correlation of $r = 0.3070$ ($p < 0.001$), and mobility is thus likely to be an additional cause. The best guess we can make is that skin is affected by at least two factors, i.e. mobility and age.

The relationships we have considered above are quite simple ones, trying to explain the apparent effect of one variable on another with the effect of a third (either in combination with, or instead of, or an as intervening factor). However, more complex relationships may hold. What if some combination of two or more other variables accounted for all the apparent relationship shown between age and skin? We can in this case test for the effect on skin by age (again we assume the relationship could not be causal the other way round, as skin deterioration could not cause our age to change) allowing for more than one other variable at once.

In fact, allowing for all the other nine variables in the Waterlow score still gives $r = 0.3276$ ($p < 0.001$) for skin and age. Thus there does seem to be a genuine effect of age on skin. This of course is a fairly trivial example as there is a wealth of evidence that skin is affected by ageing.

As a real-world example of the problems of establishing causation, consider socio-economic class and health. It is known that lower socio-economic class people are less healthy and have lower life expectancy than those in higher classes. Is it the case that being lower class causes ill-health and premature death, or is it the case (say) that lower class people are causing their own ill-health through their behaviour. Kunst et al[10] used micro data from national health interview surveys in European Union countries to examine self-reported morbidity, and used four risk-behaviour-related determinants of morbidity: tobacco and alcohol consumption, overweight and the consumption of fresh vegetables. They also used data on mortality from national longitudinal studies and 'unlinked' cross-sectional studies for 10 causes of death and three socio-economic determinants (occupational class, level of education and level of income). In every country for which data were available, morbidity rates were higher in what Kunst et al described as lower socio-economic groups. This inverse relationship held for each age group, sex, the socio-economic indicators and the morbidity indicators.[10] In every country for which data were available, they also found that mortality rates were higher among people of lower occupational classes (study of men only) and those of lower education levels. Thus it would appear that being lower class is actually bad for you. It is likely that a partial correlation of morbidity against class would show a significant result if you allowed for each of the other factors.

Another example from the real world that shows the complexity of correlation is given in several papers by Wilkinson.[11–13] Wilkinson has argued that, while poverty and mortality are correlated in a linear fashion, for the poorer countries of the world, it is not inequality of income that is the major factor, but rather the *amount of income*. This correlation breaks down above a certain value of GDP (gross domestic product) per head of population. That is, in the richer countries, the major factor associated with life expectancy is *income inequality*.

Let us now relate these results to the two aspects of correlation noted above:

- Outside a given range of values the correlation does not work. In this case above a certain value of GDP per head of population the linear relationship fails.
- The relationship between mortality and inequality of income is moderated by the level of income. At higher levels of income the correlation is substantial between mortality and income inequality, but at lower levels of income this correlation is less marked.

CONCLUSION

Correlation is the underpinning concept of many of the other techniques described in this text. It is a measure of how much one variable appears to be related to another variable. Where many variables are thought to combine to produce an effect, partial correlation is a more appropriate technique, and can allow you to uncover effects that would be hidden by simple correlation, and in particular may allow you to see spurious relationships. Correlation does not prove causation, and the results of a correlation analysis should always be used together with other information in any analysis, especially the logic of possible relationships.

EXERCISES

1. A test for correlation between GDP and infant mortality gave the following output shown below. Interpret the result, using the sign and absolute value of the correlation coefficient, and the level of significance.

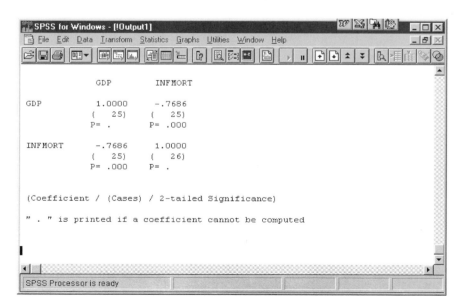

```
                  GDP           INFMORT

GDP            1.0000        -.7686
               (    25)      (    25)
               P= .          P= .000


INFMORT        -.7686         1.0000
               (    25)      (    26)
               P= .000        P= .


(Coefficient / (Cases) / 2-tailed Significance)

" . " is printed if a coefficient cannot be computed
```

2. Infant mortality and perinatal mortality in the countries used in Exercise 1 were found to be correlated (Pearson's), with $r = 0.82$ ($p = 0.001$), but a partial correlation using GDP as a controlling variable gave $r = 0.5953$ ($p = 0.002$). How would you interpret this change in the value of r and in the significance?

REFERENCES

1. Bryman A, Cramer D 1997 Quantitative data analysis. Routledge, London, p 172–180
2. Norusis M J 1993 SPSS for Windows base system user's guide. SPSS, Chicago, IL, p 291–301
3. Bryman A, Cramer D 1997 Quantitative data analysis. Routledge, London, p 196
4. Barnes J 1997. Prevention of pressure sores in community-based wheelchair users: a study examining the use of risk calculators and the relevance of risk factors to assess pressure sore risk in community-based wheelchair users. Master's Thesis, University of Birmingham, UK
5. Anthony D M, Barnes J, Unsworth J 1998 An evaluation of current risk assessment scales for decubitus ulcer in general inpatients and wheelchair users. Clinical Rehabilitation 12(2): 137–143
6. Norusis M J 1993 SPSS for Windows base system user's guide. SPSS, Chicago, IL, p 303–310
7. Bryman A, Cramer D 1997 Quantitative data analysis. Routledge, London, p 250–256
8. Bryman A, Cramer D 1997 Quantitative data analysis. Routledge, London, p 242
9. Bryman A, Cramer D 1997 Quantitative data analysis. Routledge, London, p 251
10. Kunst A E, Cavelaars A E J M, Cavelaars F, Geurts J J M, Mackenbach J P 1996 Socio-economic inequalities in morbidity and mortality in Europe: a comparative study. Department of Public Health, Erasmus University, Rotterdam
11. Wilkinson R G 1994 Health, redistribution and growth. In: A Glyn, D Miliband (eds) Paying for inequality: the economic cost of social injustice. IPPR/Rivers Oram Press, London, p 24–43
12. Wilkinson R G 1996 Unhealthy societies; the afflictions of inequality. Routledge, London, p 122
13. Wilkinson R G 1997 Health inequalities: relative or absolute material standards? British Medical Journal 7080: 314

Contingency tables

When data is at the nominal level, you are not able to use the more powerful statistical tests that assume a higher level of data (ordinal, interval or ratio). However you are often faced with questions such as 'are women more likely to develop pressure sores (does gender influence pressure sore formation)?'. This chapter describes techniques for dealing with nominal data, and goes beyond simple chi square tests as found in most introductions to statistics. In particular it deals with paired data, and with relative risk.

KEY POINTS

- Two nominal variables can be cross-tabulated to produce a table that gives the frequencies of each possible combination of values of the two variables, this is a contingency table

- The chi square (χ^2) test is a test of independence (or, equivalently, of association) of one nominal variable versus another

- Fisher's exact test can be used when the χ^2 test is inappropriate

- Paired nominal data can be tested for differences using McNemar's test

- Relative risk can be computed using nominal variables, where the likelihood of one variable given the result of another is computed

At the end of this chapter the student should be able to:

1. Use SPSS to generate the contingency tables and compute the tests for χ^2, McNemar and relative risk

2. Be able to interpret the SPSS output of the above tests

INTRODUCTION

If data are of a nominal form, you can only use quantitative analysis meaningfully by using counts and frequencies of the item, as any numerical codes applied to the items are purely labels, and cannot be analysed numerically. Rather than simply record the frequency of a given variable (say the number of nurses who smoke), we might want to compare the frequencies of more than one grouping of data (say the number of male smokers versus the number of female smokers), in which case we might have a table split by smoking habit (smoker or non-smoker) and gender (male or female). A table that gives every possible combination of frequencies is known as a *contingency table*. For an excellent review of contingency tables see the book by Everitt,[1] which gives much more detail than this chapter can hope to provide, and has numerous references to more obscure and detailed tests than he covers.

For example, in a survey of computer network sites,[2-4] the English and Scottish sites responding to the survey were as shown in Table 5.1. Suppose you wanted to compare academic sites and trusts in some way, for example their use of international networks. If Scotland were shown to use these more, it could be argued that the sample may be caused by a bias in a comparison of international networks (note that this does not imply that the sample is biased; it may correctly reflect the true proportion of academic sites, but because the Scottish proportion is different from the English figure, it may affect the comparison). If more academic sites were reported in the Scottish replies as a proportion compared with the English responses, the effect noted may be an artefact. For if academic sites use international networks more than trusts do, then the fact that the Scottish

Table 5.1 The number of English and Scottish sites that responded to the survey

Country	Number
England	262
Scotland	49
Total	311

responses reported more academic sites might explain the difference, and the geographical location had little or no real importance.

In cause and effect relationships a confounding variable is one that interferes in the direct causal relationship between the independent variable to the dependent variable.[5] In our example above we could have type of site being a confounding variable for the apparent relationship between the dependent variable (use of international networks) and the independent variable (country). In other words, it could be that the type of site is the variable that affects the use of international networks, and this confounds the apparent relationship. If this were the case, then the apparent relationship is spurious.

2 × 2 TABLES

The sites were also split into academic (90) and health trusts (257). If you split the tabular data by type of site and country you have a 2 × 2 (two rows and two columns) contingency table, as shown in Table 5.2. We make the table by taking all possible combinations of one variable against another, here country (England and Scotland) against organization (trust or academic). These tables are often referred to as *cross-tabulations*. SPSS uses this terminology, which is equivalent to calling them contingency tables.

Adding totals to the data listed in the contingency table gives Table 5.3. You can see that 17 of the 80 academic sites (21%), are Scottish compared with 32 of the 232 trusts (14%). The question to ask is whether this is a significant difference, i.e. is our sample biased? Alternatively, you could ask if the type of site and the country are *independent* of each other. If the type of organization (academic or trust) is independent of country (England

Table 5.2 The 2 × 2 contingency table for country versus organization type: England and Scotland

	NHS trusts	Academic sites
England	200 (*a*)	63 (*b*)
Scotland	32 (*c*)	17 (*d*)

Table 5.3 Contingency table for country versus organization type, with totals: England and Scotland

	NHS trusts	Academic sites	Total
England	200	63	263
Scotland	32	17	49
Total	232	80	312

or Scotland), then the proportions of each organization type should be similar for each country (and the proportion of each country represented in each organization type should be similar).

The appropriate statistical test for this contingency table is the chi square (χ^2) test, which returns a χ^2 statistic. This test looks at the difference between the expected frequencies if the variables were truly independent, and the frequencies actually observed. The test is used to assess for *independence* of the nominal data. That is, does the frequency of one category affect the frequency of another (in the present case, is the proportion of academic sites in Scotland different from the proportion of academic sites in England?) The χ^2 value may be thought of as a measure of *association* because, if two variables are found not to be independent, then it is reasonable to say that they are associated.

DEGREES OF FREEDOM

As the number of data increases, so too will any value that looks at the difference between observed and expected values. To allow for this, looking the χ^2 value up in a table it is necessary to know the number of degrees of freedom. A similar requirement is placed on many statistical tests. For χ^2 the number of degrees of freedom is given by

$$df = (r-1)(c-1)$$

where r is the number of rows and c is the number of columns in the contingency table. So for a 2×2 table df = 1, and for a 3×3 table df = 4.

The χ^2 test returns a value which, given the degrees of freedom, can be used to compute the probability (p value) that the results occurred by chance alone. A p value below the α level (typically 0.05) indicates the categories are not independent. A small section from a table of χ^2 values is shown in Table 5.4. For example if a χ^2 statistic of 4.0 was returned with one degree of freedom, then it is significant at $p < 0.05$ as it is more than 3.84, but not at the $p < 0.01$ level as it is less than 6.63. If the same statistic was associated with two degrees of freedom (say a 3×2 table), then it would not be significant even at the $p < 0.05$ level as it is less than 5.99.

Returning to the example used above, the best way to approach this problem is to ask how many of each type of site one would expect from

Table 5.4 Values of χ^2 for given degrees of freedom and α levels of 0.05 and 0.01

df	$p < 0.05$	$p < 0.01$
1	3.84	6.63
2	5.99	9.21
3	7.81	11.34
4	9.49	13.28

each country. As 263 of 311 responses were from England (84.3%), if organization type and country were independent of each other, one would expect 84.3% of the 232 health trusts and 84.3% of the 80 academic sites to be from England, or 195.6 and 67.4, respectively (all values rounded to one decimal place). Similarly, you would expect 15.7% of both total health trust and total academic sites to be from Scotland, or 34.4 and 12.6, respectively. Thus you would expect roughly 4 less English and 4 more Scottish sites than found in this survey. A similar calculation shows that 4 more academic responses from England and 4 fewer Scottish academic responses would be expected.

There is a general formula for working out expected values using the totals found for each row and column. For each cell in Table 5.3 look to the right to see the row total, and below to find the column total. For the expected value of English health trusts, the observed value (or actual value found) was 200, the row total was 263 and the column total was 232.

You can work out the expected number of responses E in each cell of the table by using the following calculation:

Equation 1: Expected values

$$E = \frac{\text{Row total} \times \text{Column total}}{\text{Overall total}}$$

Thus for English NHS trusts the expected value is (to one decimal place)

$$E = \frac{263 \times 232}{12} = 195.6$$

and for Scottish academic sites the expected value is

$$E = \frac{49 \times 80}{312} = 12.6$$

Clearly the value such as 12.6 is impossible, as sites can only exist in whole numbers (also called *integer values*; i.e. whole numbers greater than or equal to zero, e.g. 0, 1, 2, 3 but not decimal values); however, the χ^2 statistic uses non-integer values. The further the expected values are from the actual values (also called observed values) the less likely it is that the results occurred by chance alone.

Equation 2: χ^2 statistic

$$\chi^2 = \sum \frac{(O - E)^2}{E}$$

where Σ means 'sum of', i.e. for each observed and expected value work out $(O - E)^2/E$ and add them all up:

$$\chi^2 = \frac{(200 - 195.6)^2}{195.6} + \frac{(63 - 67.4)^2}{67.4} + \frac{(32 - 36.4)^2}{36.4} + \frac{(17 - 12.6)^2}{12.6}$$

$$= \frac{4.4^2}{195.6} + \frac{4.4^2}{67.4} + \frac{4.4^2}{36.4} + \frac{4.4^2}{12.6}$$

$$= 2.45$$

Note that in the case considered here (a 2×2 table) the nominator is identical (4.4^2, or 19.36) in each case. This is always true for 2×2 tables, but is not true in general. The explanation is that if there are 4.4 too many observed English health trusts this must be balanced by 4.4 too few English academic sites, and also there must be 4.4 too many Scottish academic sites to balance the shortfall in English sites, leading to the fact that there must be 4.4 too few Scottish trusts.

Equation 3: χ^2 for 2×2 tables

For the special case of a 2×2 table, χ^2 can also be computed using the formula

$$\chi^2 = \frac{N(ad - bc)^2}{(a + b)(c + d)(a + c)(b + d)}$$

where a, b, c and d are the items shown in Table 5.2. The four components of the denominator are the row and column totals.

So, for the above case

$$\chi^2 = \frac{312(200 \times 17 - 63 \times 32)^2}{(200 + 63)(32 + 17)(200 + 32)(63 + 17)}$$

$$= \frac{311 \times 1384^2}{263 \times 49 \times 232 \times 80} = 2.49$$

(*Note*: The value of 2.45 quoted above is slightly different because of rounding errors, i.e. we rounded all values to a single decimal place, which was slightly inaccurate.)

Equation 4: Yate's correction

When the numbers are small, it is advisable to use Yate's correction, which is a more conservative test. However, as Yate's correction makes very little difference as the numbers get larger, its use is advised in all cases. This involves taking 0.5 from positive discrepancies between observed and expected values, and adding 0.5 to negative discrepancies. Another way to look at this is to take 0.5 from the absolute value of any difference, which is typically shown as $|O - E|$, where the '$|$' symbol means take the value inside the symbol, and if it is negative change the sign to make it positive. Thus $|10 - 5| = |5 - 10| = 5$.

The equation used to calculate Yate's correction is

$$\chi^2 = \sum \frac{(|O - E| - 0.5)^2}{E}$$

Equation 5: Yate's correction for 2 × 2 tables

Yate's correction for the special case of a 2 × 2 table[6] can be computed as

$$\chi^2 = \frac{N(|ad - bc| - 0.5)^2}{(a + b)(c + d)(a + c)(b + d)}$$

USING SPSS TO COMPUTE χ^2

The first step to computing χ^2 is to produce contingency tables (or, as SPSS refers to them, cross-tabulations). The data are stored in two variables that are nominal. The calculation is achieved via the Statistics pull-down menu, then selecting the Summarize and then Crosstabs. You then need to state which two variables you wish to produce a table from, and put one in a column and the other in a row (it is not important which way round you do it). If this were all you did, you would get the output window shown in Figure 5.1.

The values given in Figure 5.1 are those we computed by hand above. However, we want to do more than summarize the data, we want to test for independence of the variables (i.e. to see if country affects organizational type). To do this, select Statistics from the Crosstabs dialogue box, and select Chi-square as an option. You can also elect to be shown the expected as well as observed values from the *Cells* option, in which case you will get something like the screen shown in Figure 5.2.

SPSS computes χ^2 in several ways, but the commonest variant is that devised by Pearson, which is the first line of χ^2 values given in Figure 5.2. (*Note*: This is *not* the Pearson coefficient of correlation.) All the calculations above were also done using Pearson's χ^2 value.

Pearson's χ^2 value is given (roughly 2.5) together with the significance, which here is $p = 0.11$, i.e. not significant at an α level of 0.05. Yate's continuity is shown in the second line, with a χ^2 value of about 1.97, which is also non-significant.

Note that SPSS may state the minimum expected frequency, here about

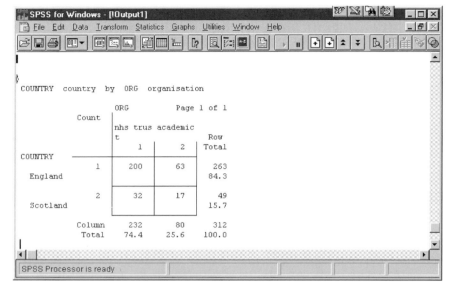

Figure 5.1 Contingency table: SPSS Output window.

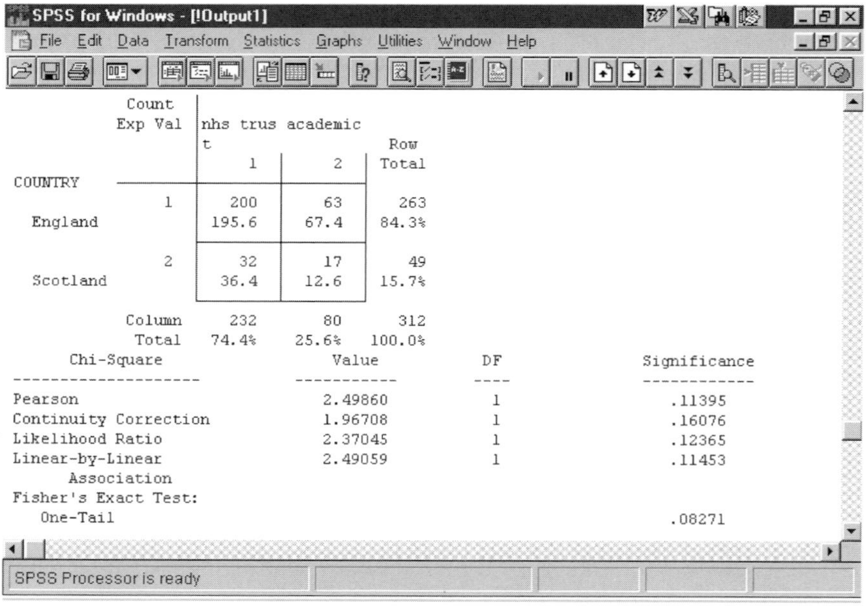

Figure 5.2 χ^2 statistic for a 2×2 contingency table: SPSS Output window.

12.6, and may in some cases report the percentage of expected frequencies below 5, both of which are indicators of a possible need to use an alternative test, i.e. Fisher's exact test (see below). Fisher's test is not indicated in Figure 5.2, but if it were you could use the value quoted.

FISHER'S EXACT TEST

If the expected values of any cell in a 2×2 table are less than 5, use of the χ^2 statistic is not recommended. (*Note*: There is some argument about the exact threshold for the expected value that is invalid for χ^2 but here we will use the conventional value of 5[7].) An alternative test is Fisher's test.

Fisher's test computes the exact probability of getting any particular set of observed values. It has been suggested that χ^2 with Yate's correction gives similar results to Fisher's exact test.[8] Fisher's exact test requires a considerable amount of calculation, and prior to the general availability of computers, χ^2 with Yate's correction might have been the preferred option. However, Fisher's test can now be easily computed, and is preferred for low figures.

Equation 6: Fisher's exact test[6]

$$P = \frac{(a + b)! \, (a + c)! \, (c + d)! \, (b + d)!}{a! \, b! \, c! \, d! \, N!}$$

where $a! = a(a - 1)(a - 2)(a - 3), \ldots, 1$; for example, $4! = 4 \times 3 \times 2 \times 1 = 24$.

This is the probability of getting exactly the figures found. In practice we would usually want to know whether at least the figure found for, say, academic Welsh sites (Table 5.5) was what we would expect, so if we found five academic Welsh sites, and this was less than we were expecting, what would be the likelihood of getting 5 or less. Thus the probability of 5, 4, 3, 2, 1 and no sites could be calculated and added together. Fisher's test returns a p value, and the interpretation is similar to χ^2: a low p value indicates that the categories are not independent.

For example, if Wales and Northern Ireland were compared in the survey, and the smaller numbers listed in Table 5.5 were obtained, then

Table 5.5 Contingency table for country versus organization type, with totals: Northern Ireland and Wales

Country	NHS trusts	Academic sites	Total
Wales	14	5	19
Northern Ireland	9	4	13
Total	23	9	32

$$P = \frac{19!\ 23!\ 13!\ 9!}{14!\ 5!\ 9!\ 4!\ 32!} = 0.296$$

The above calculation is greatly facilitated by using a powerful calculator, a spreadsheet program or a statistics package.

We have computed the probability of getting exactly five academic and 14 NHS Welsh sites, and four and nine academic and NHS Northern Irish sites respectively. But what we want to know is not whether we could have got exactly five academic sites, but what is the probability of getting five or less (this is the same as asking whether we could get 14 or more NHS trusts). Thus if $P(5)$ is the probability of getting exactly five Welsh academic sites, we do not want $P(5)$ so much as the sum of all possible arrangements where the number is five or less, i.e. $P(5)$, $P(4)$, $P(3)$, $P(2)$, $P(1)$ and $P(0)$. Adding all these together will give the probability of getting five or less Welsh academic sites.

If there were four Welsh academic sites, and the totals were the same, then there would need to be 15 Welsh health trusts (Table 5.6). But also the number of Northern Irish academic sites would need to decrease to eight, and NHS sites increase to five to keep the column and row totals the same. The above formula would give a $P(4) = 0.178$, and, continuing, $P(3) = 0.06$, $P(2) = 0.01$, $P(1) = 0.0009$ and $P(0) = 0.00003$ (to one significant place), and adding gives an overall value of $p = 0.54$ (to two decimal places). In other words, more than 50% of the time we could get these figures by chance alone, so we cannot reject the null hypothesis that the two variables show no significant dependence on each other.

However, we did not really need to compute more than the first value, $P(5)$, because a value of around 0.30 means there is a 30% chance we could have got these exact values by chance alone, and therefore the values appear to be independent of each other even without going further and adding the other probabilities.

SPSS would have given the data shown in Figure 5.3. Note that Fisher's test considers the values at or below a given value (or at and above), and thus it is one-tailed. Sometimes (when the sample size in each group is the same) a two-tailed Fisher's test is meaningful, but in general this is not the case and the one-tailed test should be quoted. (The two-tailed test (see Fig. 5.3) can be interpreted as giving the probability that there are 5 or less

Table 5.6   Contingency table for country versus organization type with totals: Wales and Northern Ireland

	NHS trusts	Academic sites	Total
Wales	15	4	19
Northern Ireland	8	5	13
Total	23	9	32

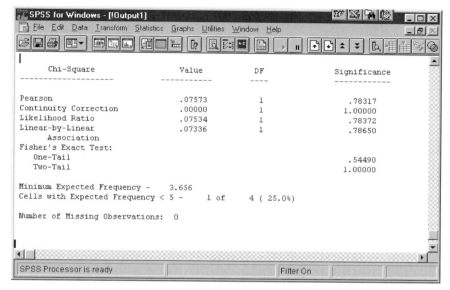

```
  SPSS for Windows - [!Output1]                                          _ □ ×
  File  Edit  Data  Transform  Statistics  Graphs  Utilities  Window  Help        _ 8 ×

  │
      Chi-Square                      Value          DF            Significance
  -------------------              -----------      ----          ------------

  Pearson                            .07573          1                .78317
  Continuity Correction              .00000          1               1.00000
  Likelihood Ratio                   .07534          1                .78372
  Linear-by-Linear                   .07336          1                .78650
      Association
  Fisher's Exact Test:
      One-Tail                                                        .54490
      Two-Tail                                                       1.00000

  Minimum Expected Frequency -    3.656
  Cells with Expected Frequency < 5 -     1 of      4 ( 25.0%)

  Number of Missing Observations:   0

  │
  ◄ │ │                                                                    ►

  SPSS Processor is ready                        │         Filter On
```

Figure 5.3   Fisher's test: SPSS Output window.

Welsh health trust sites or more than 6, which will clearly always be the case, and is trivially 100% likely.)

$\chi^2 \, r \times c$

The 2×2 table is a particularly simple case. Let us now look at the full table for all four countries, as shown in Table 5.7. The expected values can be computed using Equation 1. For example,

$$E(\text{England, NHS trusts}) \qquad\qquad = \frac{263 \times 255}{344} = 195.0$$

$$E(\text{England, academic sites}) \qquad\quad = \frac{263 \times 89}{344} = 68.0$$

$$E(\text{Northern Ireland, NHS trusts}) \quad = \frac{13 \times 254}{344} = 9.6$$

$$E(\text{Northern Ireland, academic sites}) = \frac{13 \times 89}{344} = 3.4$$

Note that the expected values for England add up to 263, and those for Northern Ireland add to 13, as they should.

While you can compute this by hand, if the data are stored in SPSS as the variables ORG and COUNTRY, then using the method above, SPSS

Table 5.7 Contingency table for country versus organization type, with totals: all UK countries

Country	NHS trusts	Academic sites	Total
England	200	63	263
Scotland	32	17	49
Wales	14	5	19
Northern Ireland	9	4	13
Total	255	89	344

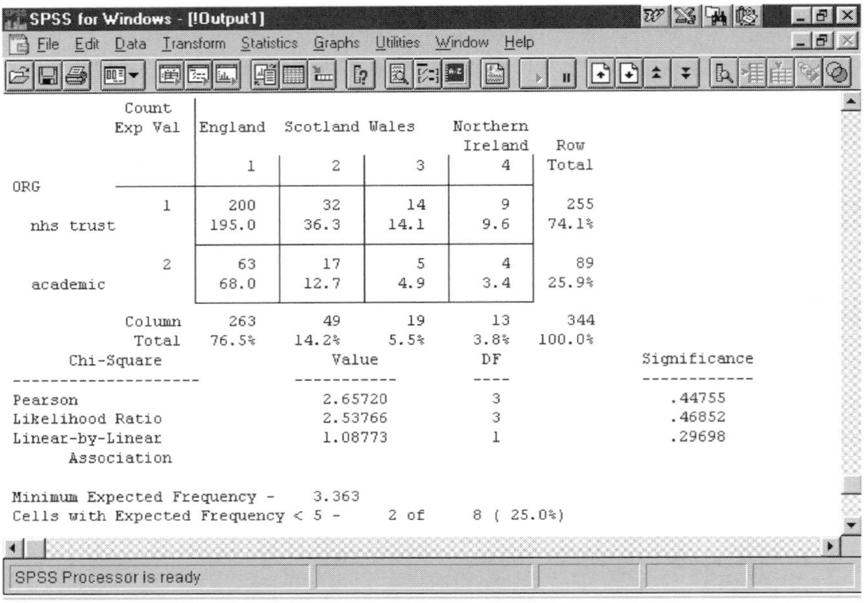

```
 SPSS for Windows - [!Output1]

 File  Edit  Data  Transform  Statistics  Graphs  Utilities  Window  Help

            Count
            Exp Val   England  Scotland Wales    Northern
                                                 Ireland   Row
                         1        2        3        4      Total
 ORG
               1       200       32       14        9        255
      nhs trust        195.0    36.3     14.1      9.6      74.1%

               2        63       17        5        4         89
      academic         68.0     12.7      4.9      3.4      25.9%

            Column     263       49       19       13        344
            Total      76.5%    14.2%     5.5%     3.8%    100.0%
         Chi-Square            Value              DF         Significance
 --------------------        ----------         ----       ------------
 Pearson                       2.65720            3            .44755
 Likelihood Ratio             2.53766            3            .46852
 Linear-by-Linear             1.08773            1            .29698
         Association

 Minimum Expected Frequency -    3.363
 Cells with Expected Frequency < 5 -    2 of    8 ( 25.0%)

 SPSS Processor is ready
```

Figure 5.4 χ^2 statistic for a 2×4 contingency table: SPSS Output window.

would report as shown in Figure 5.4. Note that the expected frequencies equate with our manual calculations. The p value (shown as significance on this Output screen) is not at all significant. Note that Fisher's exact test has not been calculated, as it is only appropriate for 2×2 tables, and so we must look at χ^2 calculations. However, with one minimum expected frequency over 3 and another of 4.9, using a rigid criterion of more than 20% expected frequencies < 5, the χ^2 statistic is inappropriate. Just a slight relaxation of the criterion allows the test to be used.

CORRELATED DATA

The χ^2 statistic is a measure of independence of nominal variables, and assumes that the data have been collected independently. There are

Table 5.8 Contingency table for health trusts with strategic policy versus those with training programme

With strategic policy on networks	With computer network training Yes	No
No	24 (a)	102 (b)
Yes	61 (c)	70 (d)

occasions when we want to measure differences for *paired* data. This assumes that the data are correlated, in which case the standard χ^2 test is not appropriate. In particular, if we have matched data, or repeated measures on the same subject, we are not permitted to use the standard χ^2 test. An example might be if we wanted to know if those health trusts that had a written policy on computer networks were equally likely to have training in place for their staff. We might get figures like those shown in Table 5.8.

The number of trusts with both policy or training and the number with neither policy or training do not tell us much about the differences between the organizations. But if computer training and written policies were present in the same proportions, you would expect there to be as many trusts with no policy but with training (in this case 24) as those with no training but with policy (here 70). The difference between these two figures gives some indication of whether the two variables are independent of each other.

It can be shown that a χ^2 statistic, *McNemar's test*, can be computed[9] as follows:

$$\chi^2 = \frac{(a-d)^2}{(a+d)}$$

where a and d correspond to the values shown in the table that have one attribute but not the other.

In fact a correction can be made for continuity (for the same reason that Yate's correction is made), and the formula becomes[9]

$$\chi^2 = \frac{(|a-d|-1)^2}{(a+d)}$$

So, for the above case

$$\chi^2 = \frac{(|24-70|-1)^2}{24+70} = \frac{45^2}{94} = 21.54$$

which is highly significant ($p < 0.0001$), which indicates that there is a difference in the proportions of those trusts that have training and those that have policies; there are significantly less trusts with training than with a strategic policy.

To compute McNemar's test in SPSS, select Non-parametric Tests from the Statistics pull-down menu, and then click on Two Related Samples. You will be asked to give the two test variables, and select *McNemar* as the test (there are other related sample tests in this section of SPSS, but they require ordinal data).

McNemar is often used before and after experiments, in a similar fashion as the Wilcoxon or the paired Student's *t*-test might be used on (at least) ordinal data or normally distributed (typically interval/ratio) data, respectively.

RELATIVE RISK

Suppose that one nominal variable is present and you want to work out how likely it is that the other one will be so too. We can think of the *risk* of getting a positive response for one given a positive response for the other. Suppose we wanted to know how likely it is that an organization has a written policy given its type of organization (trust or academic) (Table 5.9). The proportion of those academic organizations that have a policy is

$$\frac{a}{a + b} = \frac{55}{55 + 202} = 0.214$$

(to three decimal places), and the corresponding proportion for trusts is

$$\frac{c}{c + d} = \frac{17}{17 + 70} = 0.195$$

Thus the *relative risk* Ψ of an academic organization having a written policy compared with that of a trust is $\Psi = 0.214/0.195 = 1.097$, and for trusts compared with academic organizations is $\Psi = 0.195/0.214 = 0.911$, which means that the 'risk' of a trust having a written policy is about 91% that of an academic site. (*Note*: The term 'risk' is used as we are often looking at the chance of a disease occurring in some group, although in

Table 5.9 Contingency table for academic site versus written policy

Academic site	With written policy	
	Yes	No
Yes	55 (*a*)	202 (*b*)
No	17 (*c*)	70 (*d*)

this case the 'risk' more naturally means the chance of a policy being present.)

If the number of organizations that are positive for the condition a and c (i.e. have a policy; but this could be having a disease in another example) is few compared with the overall number $a + b$ and $a + c$, then the risks become approximately a/b and c/d. The relative risk becomes

$$\frac{a\,|\,b}{c\,|\,d} = \frac{ad}{bc}$$

This is referred to as the *odds ratio* and is an approximation to the relative risk. In the present case we could have $\Psi = (55\times70)/(202\times17) = 1.12$ (this is slightly different to the value above because of the approximation used) for the increased chance of academic organizations having a policy, or 0.892 for the reduced chance of trusts having a policy.

However, is this increased chance of academic organizations having a policy significant? This can be determined using a formula for the *95% confidence interval* (CI):[10]

$$95\% \text{ CI} = \text{ln } \Psi \pm 1.96\sqrt{\text{var (ln } \Psi)}$$

where var (ln Ψ) can be shown to be $(1/a + 1/b + 1/c + 1/d)$, which here would be $0.019 + 0.005 + 0.06 + 0.014 = 0.098$. So

$$\text{ln } \Psi \pm 1.96 \sqrt{\text{var(ln } \Psi)} = -0.115 \pm 0.61 = [-0.725, 0.495]$$

or, after taking exponentials the range is [0.48, 1.64]. This means that the 95% confidence interval for the risk is between 0.48 and 1.64 (48% and 164%). This range includes 1.0 (100%), which means it is quite likely that there is no increased 'risk' of an academic site having a policy.

To use SPSS to compute relative risk, use the same sequence as for χ^2 (select Statistics pull-down menu, then Summarize, then Crosstabs) and then click on Statistics in the dialogue box, again as for Chi square, but this time select Risk rather than Chi-square. You would get the output screen shown in Figure 5.5. (Note that the rows and columns contain the same information, but in a slightly different order, as Table 5.9). In SPSS, the odds ratio is given as Case Control.

The above example may be seen as a little contrived. A more natural example provided by mortality tables. Here we will use mortality figures derived from source material provided by the World Health Organization (WHO). (*Note*: The analyses, interpretations and conclusions are those of the author. The survivor data are computed from population figures rounded to the nearest 100 with exact death figures subtracted from

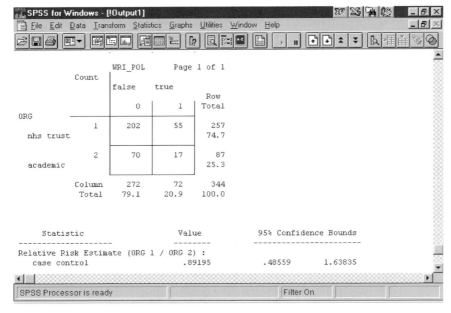

Figure 5.5 Relative risk: SPSS Output window.

Table 5.10 Mortality data for Latvian men and women aged 55–59 years

	Died	Survived
Males	2061	66 339
Females	878	85 662

them.) Specifically, let us compare the mortality of males against that of females for Latvia in 1993 for the age group 55–59 years (Table 5.10). The odds ratio for males versus females is:

$$\frac{2061 \times 85\,662}{878 \times 66\,339} = 3.03$$

(to two decimal places). That is Latvian males aged 55–59 years are more than three times as likely to die than are females of the same age.

If the 95% confidence limits are put in we get

$$\text{var (In } \Psi) = \frac{1}{2061} + \frac{1}{66\,339} + \frac{1}{878} + \frac{1}{85\,662} = 0.00165$$

$$\Psi = \frac{2061 \times 85\,662}{878 \times 66\,339} = 3.03$$

$$\text{In } \Psi = 1.11$$
$$\text{In } \Psi \pm 1.96\sqrt{\text{var (In } \Psi)} = 1.11 \pm 1.96\sqrt{0.001\,65}$$
$$= 1.11 \pm 0.080$$
$$= [1.03,1.18]$$

(all values to three significant places). On taking exponentials, this becomes [2.80,3.25]. So we are 95% confident that the lowest odds ratio is 2.80 and the highest is 3.25; in either event men are about three times as likely to die as women.

It is in fact universal that men die more than women in this age band (and most others), although this is a particularly high ratio. Men of the same age in Sweden, for example (Table 5.11), have an odds ratio of 1.83 with a 95% confidence level of [1.70,1.98]; i.e. at most, Swedish men are about twice as likely to die in this age band as are Swedish women.

A further comparison we can make is one between the mortality of Swedish and Latvian men (Table 5.12). The data give an odds ratio that is greatly in excess of what you would expect for two neighbouring European countries (in fact Latvia has shown a massive rise in death rates, especially for males in the young and middle age ranges):

$$\frac{2061 \times 210\,284}{1716 \times 66\,339} = 3.81$$

Table 5.11 Mortality data for Swedish men and women aged 55–59 years

	Died	Survived
Males	1716	210 284
Females	976	219 024

Table 5.12 Mortality data for Swedish and Latvian men aged 55–59 years

	Died	Survived
Latvia	2061	66 339
Sweden	1716	210 284

(to two decimal places). That is, Latvian men aged 55–59 years are almost four times as likely to die as are Swedish men of the same age.

If the 95% confidence limits are put in we get

$$\text{var (ln } \Psi) = \frac{1}{2061} + \frac{1}{66\ 339} + \frac{1}{1716} + \frac{1}{210\ 284} = 0.001\ 09$$

$\Psi = 3.81$
$\ln \Psi = 1.34$
$$\ln \Psi \pm 1.96\sqrt{\text{var (ln } \Psi)} = 1.34 \pm 1.96\ \sqrt{0.001\ 09}$$
$$= 1.34 \pm 0.06$$
$$= [1.28, 1.40]$$

(all values to three significant places). On taking exponentials, this becomes [3.60,4.06]. Thus Latvian men in this age band are between about three and a half and four times as likely to die as are Swedish men in the same band.

OTHER AREAS

Some areas not covered by this text, but which are described in fuller texts such as the one by Everitt,[1] include:

- *Correspondence analysis*: the use of biplots to graphically show relationships among categorical variables
- *Combining tables*: where many tables from (say) different geographical regions may be combined to give larger values in each cell, which gives increased power, when this is appropriate
- *Multidimensional tables*: we have concentrated on two-way splits of data (e.g. organization type by country), but there is no reason why this cannot be extended to three-way or greater splits.

The reader is referred to Everitt[1] for these and other more complex uses of contingency tables.

EXERCISES

1. The two variables of sore formation (1 = sore, 0 = no sore) and sex (0 = male, 1 = female) can be cross-tabulated as shown below, where the expected values are below the actual values. Interpert the output of the χ^2 test.

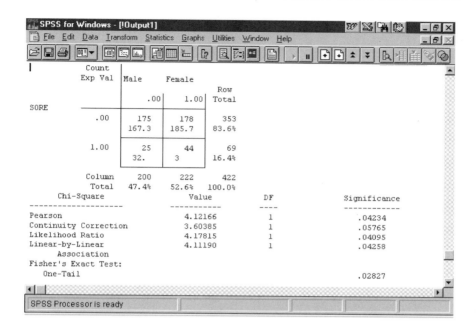

2. Running the relative risk test on the same data as in Exercise 1 gives the data shown below. Interpret the result.

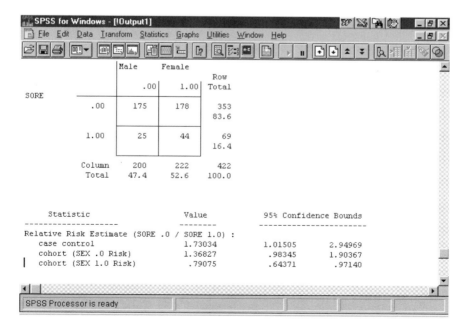

REFERENCES

1. Everitt B S 1992 The analysis of contingency tables. Chapman & Hall, London, p 14
2. Anthony D M 1996 A survey of computer network usage in NHS trusts. Health Informatics 2(4): 199–205
3. Anthony D M 1997 A comparative study of computer networks in the NHS and the academic sector of the UK. Nursing Standard 11(18): 34–38
4. Anthony D M 1997 The value of computer networks in nursing. Professional Nurse 12(12): 865–868
5. Dempsey P A, Dempsey A D 1996 Nursing research: text and workbook. Little, Brown, Boston, MA, p 226
6. Everitt B S 1992 The analysis of contingency tables. Chapman & Hall, London, p 14
7. Everitt B S 1992 The analysis of contingency tables. Chapman & Hall, London, p 39
8. Everitt B S 1992 The analysis of contingency tables. Chapman & Hall, London, p 18
9. Everitt B S 1992 The analysis of contingency tables. Chapman & Hall, London, p 20
10. Everitt B S 1992 The analysis of contingency tables. Chapman & Hall, London, p 31

Analysis of variance (ANOVA) and multiple ANOVA

This chapter explores differences between group means. We start with a simple case of two groups, extend the argument to many groups, and then to more complicated experimental designs, such as assessing differences among many groups for many dependent variables simultaneously. Similarly, the concept of paired data (which could be compared using the paired Student's t-test) is extended to three or more related variables (say three serial blood tests on a patient). For a readable but extensive text on ANOVA, including repeated measures, the reader is referred to Hand & Taylor.[1]

KEY POINTS

- ANOVA is a parametric technique: it assumes normality

- A non-parametric equivalent of ANOVA is the Kruskal–Wallis test

- Student's *t*-test for independent groups is equivalent to ANOVA with two groups

- ANOVA tests for differences between groups

- ANOVA assumes one dependent variable, and one or more independent categorical variables

- ANOVA allows analysis of data using very sophisticated experimental designs

- Transformation of non-normal data to normal data is sometimes appropriate, and allows more powerful analysis

- An extension of ANOVA to multiple dependent variables is multiple analysis of variance (MANOVA)

- Repeated-measures ANOVA can be used on more than two related variables

At the end of this chapter the student should be able to:

1. Determine the conditions under which ANOVA is appropriate

2. Determine if the data are normally distributed

3. Interpret the output from SPSS for the Student's t-test

4. Set up SPSS appropriately for a given ANOVA design

5. Interpret the output from SPSS for one way ANOVA, factorial designs and repeated-measures ANOVA

6. State when MANOVA is appropriate in preference to ANOVA

7. Interpret the output from SPSS for MANOVA for several dependent variables and several factors

GROUP DIFFERENCES

Example: examination results

This example is taken from the research proposal and dissertation by Victoria Naughten.[2]

In a nursing school in the West Midlands, UK, there is a 4-year nursing degree programme. This programme has a common foundation for 2 years, and then the students split into three branches: adult nursing, child health and mental health. Students continue to take combined lectures and assignments (management, research methods and statistics, etc.), but also specialized branch subjects, where they are assessed separately.

It is necessary, to satisfy the examinations board, to ensure that the branches are marked consistently, so that students in each branch are given an equal chance of obtaining a good degree classification. It is also required that consistency across years is maintained, i.e. the degree does not get harder or easier from one year to another. Personal tutors also want to know whether their individual students are gaining similar marks in each year, i.e. does a good mark in year one result (typically) in similar marks in other years.

This raises the following problems, which this chapter will analyse:

- Are the marks significantly different from year to year?
- Is the marking significantly different from branch to branch?
- Are the marks from a cohort of students statistically different in each year?

Two groups

Suppose we only have complete marks for the 1991 and 1992 intakes, but marks are available for 1993 and 1994 in part (the course has not yet been completed). The marks for the two different years 1991 and 1992 can be compared to see if the overall scores obtained by successive years are similar. If there is a big difference there are two possible explanations: the students were genuinely better in one year, or the assessment was harder, in one year.

If you wanted to test the significance of the difference between two independent groups with respect to some variable at the ordinal, interval or ratio level, there are two main statistical tests you can use:

- *Student's independent groups* t-*test*. This is appropriate if the data are normally distributed and the variances in the two groups are roughly equal. This usually implies interval or ratio data, but if ordinal data are found to be normally distributed a parametric test such as Student's t-test is appropriate.
- *Mann–Whitney test*. This is appropriate if the conditions for Student's t-test do not apply.

Since Student's t-test requires normal distributions, the *Kolmogorov–Smirnov goodness of fit test*, which can be used to assess normality (available in SPSS under the pull-down menu Statistics, then Nonparametric Tests, then 1 sample K-S) is applied. If 'final' is the variable name for the final degree mark, then selecting this variable, and allowing the default distribution of normal to be tested (the Kolmogorov–Smirnov test can also test for two other distributions), the display shown in Figure 6.1 is seen.

The Kolmogorov–Smirnov goodness of fit test output (Fig. 6.1) shows that the hypothesis that the sample came from a normal distribution could not be rejected ($p = 0.38$). Another method of checking for normality is to plot a histogram (Fig. 6.2). Further evidence is that the mean, median (the middle value) and mode (the most frequent observation) of the data should be roughly the same in a normal distribution. In our example, the mean is 61.1 and the median is 61.8, so they are similar, although not identical (the mode here is actually of little interest, as all values are unique except one (58.85), which occurred twice). Therefore, even though from inspection the distribution looks slightly skewed, it is possible to use a parametric test such as Student's t-test. Choosing the pull-down menu Statistics, and

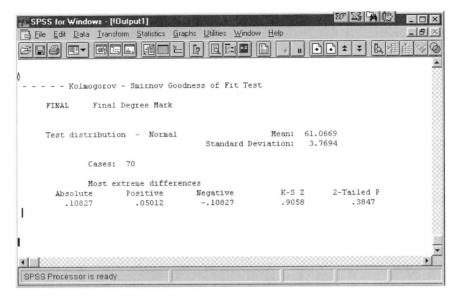

Figure 6.1 Kolmogorov–Smirnov goodness of fit test: SPSS Output screen.

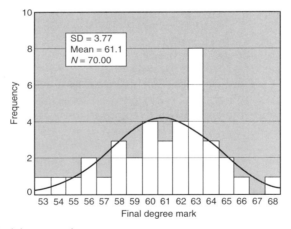

Figure 6.2 Final degree marks.

selecting Compare Means and then Independent Samples T Test, with year as the grouping variable, gives the output shown in Figure 6.3.

Figure 6.3 is possibly confusing, so let us go through it line by line. The mean, standard deviation (SD) and standard error (SE) for each year (group) are given. As the data are assumed to be normally distributed and in a normal distribution 95% of values lie within 1.96 standard deviations of

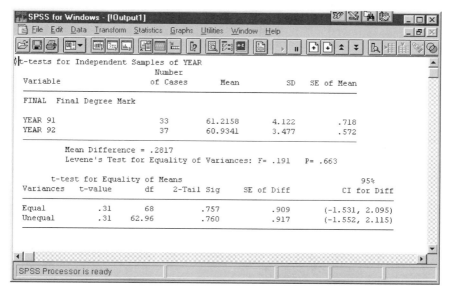

Figure 6.3   Student's *t*-tests for independent samples of year: SPSS Output screen.

the mean we can say, for example, that in the year 1991 (SD = 4.1) 95% of students gained marks in the range 61.2 ± 8.2 (rounding all values to one decimal place). Then we are told that the mean difference is about 0.28, i.e. the mean of year 1991 is about 0.28 more than that of 1992.

But the *t*-test assumes that the variance is similar, so a test is needed to check this. *Levene's test* is employed, and shows (*p* = 0.67) that the null hypothesis, i.e. that the variances are similar, can be accepted; so we can proceed. The *P* value reported from Levene's test is *not* the significance of the *t*-test (a common misconception). The *t* value for 68 degrees of freedom is given, (*t* = 0.31), but it is the *p* value we really care about. Finally, the significance of the *t*-test (the *p* value), assuming equal variance (here a reasonable assumption, as Levene's test is not significant), shows that *p* = 0.76, so we can accept the null hypothesis, i.e. there is no significant difference between the groups. Note that we use a two-tailed test, as we do not make any assumption that one year will necessarily be higher scoring than the other (we are as interested in knowing if year 1992 is higher than 1991 as we are in whether 1991 is higher than 1992). An alternative way of expressing the significance of the result is to say that the 95% confidence interval (CI) for the difference of the means contains zero, i.e. the mean values are the same. Some people find this concept confusing, but clearly if there is more than a 5% chance that the difference between the means of the groups is zero, then at the 5% threshold we are not able to state that the means found are significantly different. The 95% CI is -1.531 to $+2.095$, which does indeed contain zero, so the groups are not significantly different at the conventional 5% level.

So if the students of 1992 complain that they have been unfairly treated we can show evidence that the marking overall is similar to that in 1991 (not identical, 1992 does score slightly lower), and as the students in both years were selected on the basis of similar criteria (entry A levels) the two groups were probably similar academically. Therefore, the assessments are probably consistent, if not fair.

More than two groups

The nurses are all marked together in years one and two, but in years three and four they separate into three branches (adult nursing, mental health and child health), with some shared modules. Suppose one branch (say the child health branch) decided that they were being disadvantaged compared with the other two branches. One could perform the relevant test for two groups for every possible combination (in this case three: adult nursing versus mental health, adult nursing versus child health, mental health versus child health), but there are two problems with this:

• The number of combinations increases rapidly as the number of groups increase. For example, two groups have only one possible pair, three groups have three pairs, and four groups have 12 pairs.

• Multiple pairwise testing results in several significance tests being carried out, one for each pair. It is not appropriate to treat each of these as a single test using the conventional 5% level of significance; because there are multiple tests, the probability in any single test of finding a significant result by chance is no longer 0.05 (5 out of 100). A more conservative p value is required for each pairwise test. As Glantz[3] has pointed out, if multiple comparisons are made, a conservative estimate of the multiple test p value is obtained by adding the p values of the individual tests together. The use of the Bonferroni inequality (whereby the revised α value for multiple comparisons is obtained by dividing the required α value for a single test, assumed here to be 0.05, by the number of comparisons) is recommended by MacArthur & Jackson,[4] although they note that this is too conservative a test if the number of pairwise comparisons is greater than five.

The solution is to use a different test, for parametric data the analysis of variance (ANOVA) is the appropriate test. ANOVA is an extension of the t-test, and for two groups it is identical to the t-test. Student's t-test looks at whether the difference between two groups is explicable by the variance within each group. If two groups with a small difference between their mean values show a large variance, the distributions will largely overlap, and it is less likely that the observed difference is significant. Conversely, if two groups have the same mean difference but a smaller variance, there is a smaller overlap and we are more likely to consider the groups as being genuinely different (Fig. 6.4).

Figure 6.4a shows the curves for two groups that differ by a small amount in mean value, but overlap almost completely due to the large variance of each group. It would be difficult to be sure that the difference in the mean value did not occur by chance. For any given value it is not possible to say with any certainty to which group it belongs. The curves in Figure 6.4b show an identical difference in mean value as those in Figure 6.4a, but do not overlap at all due to the much smaller variance. It is much less likely that these two groups would have occurred by chance; if you knew the value of a given datum point, you could say with certainty which group it came from.

ONE-WAY ANOVA

ANOVA looks at the variance of several means (for different groups) and

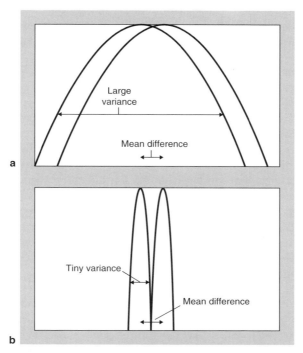

Figure 6.4 Curves (smoothed histograms) for four groups: (a) a pair of groups that show large variances; (b) a pair of groups that show small variances. The difference in the mean values of the two groups is the same in (a) and (b).

works out whether the variance within each group is high enough to account for the differences noted between the groups. If individual groups have a very high variance, then the means of randomly selected groups will tend to vary more than if the groups had very small individual variances. Thus a ratio (the F ratio) of the two variances, between group and within group, is a measure of how likely the groups are to be randomly selected from the same population. Looking at it the other way around, if we have several distinct groups, we would expect them not to show between-group variances that could be explained by purely random effects, but if we do find this to be the case then the groups cannot be presumed to have any real effect on the measured variable.

In 1992 one of the course branches (child health) was indeed noted to be marked harder than the other two; the mean score for the child health branch was about 56, while those for the adult nursing and mental health branches were about 61 and 65, respectively. Could these marks have occurred by chance? The examination mark under question was the first of two in the third year, and is labelled BRAN1_3.

Choosing the Statistics pull-down menu in SPSS, we select Compare Means and then One-Way ANOVA. One-Way ANOVA assumes we have a Factor, which is the group variable (typically a nominal variable) and a Dependent Variable, which will typically be at the interval/ratio level, although an ordinal variable that is approximately normally distributed might be used. If we choose 'branch' as Factor and BRAN1_3 as Dependent Variable, we get the output shown in Figure 6.5.

ANOVA tests the null hypothesis that the different groups have the same mean value. It returns an F ratio and a probability (p value) that the given F value could be obtained by chance. The important items to note are the F value and its significance. The F value increases as the groups differ more, so a low value indicates little or no real difference and an increasingly high value indicates an increasingly real difference. In addition, the more data that are analysed the higher the F value. Thus, as with many other tests, the test result needs to be calibrated against the amount of data, which is usually measured by the *degrees of freedom*. SPSS does the equivalent of looking up in a table for a given F-test statistic and a corresponding number of degrees of freedom, returning a p value which it names F Prob. (*Note*: In other ANOVA modules this is referred to as Sig of F. SPSS has little consistency in labelling of significance.)

The Output screen in Figure 6.5 shows a p value of 0.001, so the likelihood of obtaining this F ratio by chance is remote. Thus we can conclude that the null hypothesis that the branches have no significant difference with respect to the mark BRAN1_3 should be rejected, i.e. the branches do seem to be significantly different with respect to branch.

However, which groups are different? Is it the case that two groups are similar but both different to the third? If so, which one? Or is it the case

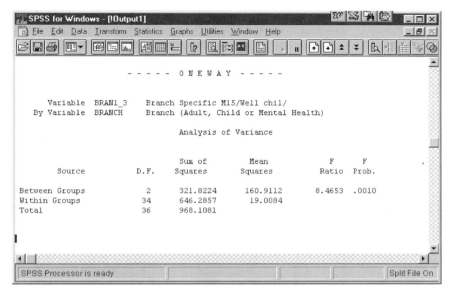

Figure 6.5 One-way ANOVA: SPSS Output screen.

that all groups are significantly different from each other? We could perform Student's *t*-test on each pair but, as stated above, this is not acceptable as we are likely to produce type I errors, and as the number of groups increases a large number of tests need to be undertaken. There are specific tests for determining the significance of pairwise tests. These are known as *post hoc tests*. SPSS offers a choice of such tests, each of which has advantages and disadvantages. *Sheffé's test* is a commonly used test of this type. If we select this test in the Post-Hoc dialogue box we get the display shown in Figure 6.6.

The Output box in Figure 6.6 gives a display that compares each group with all other groups. It is a bit like the mileage charts you see in map books that show the distance between each town to all other towns. First, SPSS tells us which post hoc test we have selected, and the algorithm used to determine if two groups are different. Then it displays all the possible combinations, with an asterisk (*) indicating each significant pairwise comparison. Thus there is no significant difference between group 1 (adult nursing) and group 3 (mental health), but the differences between group 2 (child health) and both of the two other groups are significant. So, although mental health scores are lower than adult nursing, the difference is not significant (i.e. the different mean scores could easily have occurred by chance), but the child health branch does score significantly lower than both of the other two groups.

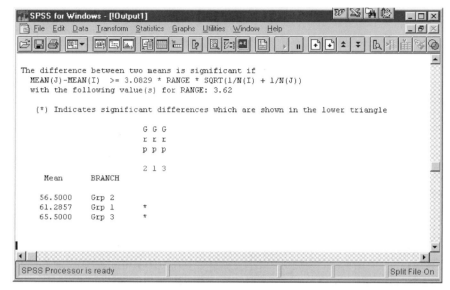

Figure 6.6 One-way ANOVA, Scheffé's test: SPSS Output screen.

ANOVA USING COVARIATES

One of the possible reason why students in the child-health branch did less well could be that they were poorer students. If this is the case we might expect them to do less well on (say) the research course, which is not branch specific. ANOVA allows us to put in the research score as a *covariate*. The idea here is that if the research score (not marked by the child health team) predicts the child health score (which is marked by the child health team) then there is no reason to believe that the child health team are marking more severely than the other two teams. In this case the two marks would be correlated. The covariate approach allows for any correlation between two variables and then gives an ANOVA result, having allowed for any correlation. In other words, it removes the effect of the covariate variable.

In SPSS, ANOVA using covariates is accessed through the Generalized Linear Model, MANOVA – General Factorial menu. The Output screen shown in Figure 6.7 uses the research mark in the same year (year three) to remove any overall differences in student marks as measured by the research score before calculating the ANOVA for the BRAN1_3 mark as the dependent variable and BRANCH as the factor. A regression analysis is done to calculate the variance that is due to the covariate, and any variance left is considered to be possibly due to the effect of branch. It can be seen that even after allowing for the research mark the *p* value is 0.01.

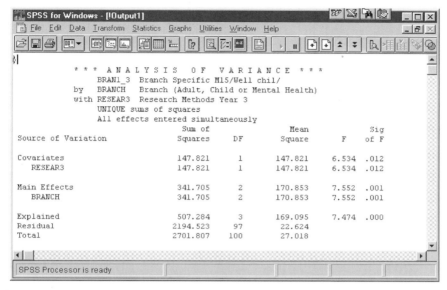

Figure 6.7   ANOVA using covariates: SPSS Output screen.

This is despite the research mark being significant as a source of variance since the p value is 0.012. The conclusion we are permitted to draw is that the overall ability of the students (as measured by the research score) does not account for the differences seen.

MANOVA

So far we have concentrated on calculating the differences in one variable. However, there are many marks to explore in the course, and we would now like to find out whether the students on the child health branch are disadvantaged throughout the course. We could do several ANOVA analyses, one for each score, but again we would run into type I error problems. It is preferable to use a different technique, and to explore the significance of all variables of interest simultaneously; this is called *multiple ANOVA*, or MANOVA. In MANOVA the significances of any differences are reported in one test. In SPSS this is achieved by selecting the Multivariate option from the ANOVA Models option in the Statistics pull-down menu. The dialogue box is similar to the one for ANOVA, except that you can select more than one dependent variable. If we selected six marks and the final year marks, we would get the Output box shown in Figure 6.8.

Note that only one mark, BRAN1_3, is seen as significant, although CHILD2 approaches significance, the latter being a mark for the child

EFFECT .. BRANCH
Multivariate Tests of Significance (S = 2, M = 2 , N = 29 1/2)

Test Name	Value	Approx. F	Hypoth. DF	Error DF	Sig. of F
Pillais	.36787	1.99636	14.00	124.00	.023
Hotellings	.45434	1.94717	14.00	120.00	.028
Wilks	.66500	1.97189	14.00	122.00	.025
Roys	.21496				

Note.. F statistic for WILKS' Lambda is exact.

EFFECT .. BRANCH (Cont.)
Univariate F-tests with (2,67) D. F.

Variable	Hypoth. SS	Error SS	Hypoth. MS	Error MS	F	Sig. of F
BIOL2	57.71925	1727.26646	28.85963	25.78010	1.11945	.332
BRAN1_3	178.69317	1573.59255	89.34658	23.48646	3.80417	.027
CHILD2	81.90807	1051.86335	40.95404	15.69945	2.60863	.081
FINAL	19.16023	961.23228	9.58012	14.34675	.66776	.516
MENTAL2	12.58137	1391.26149	6.29068	20.76510	.30295	.740
PHYSILL2	19.43851	1345.76149	9.71925	20.08599	.48388	.619
RESEAR3	99.85108	2567.28263	49.92554	38.31765	1.30294	.279

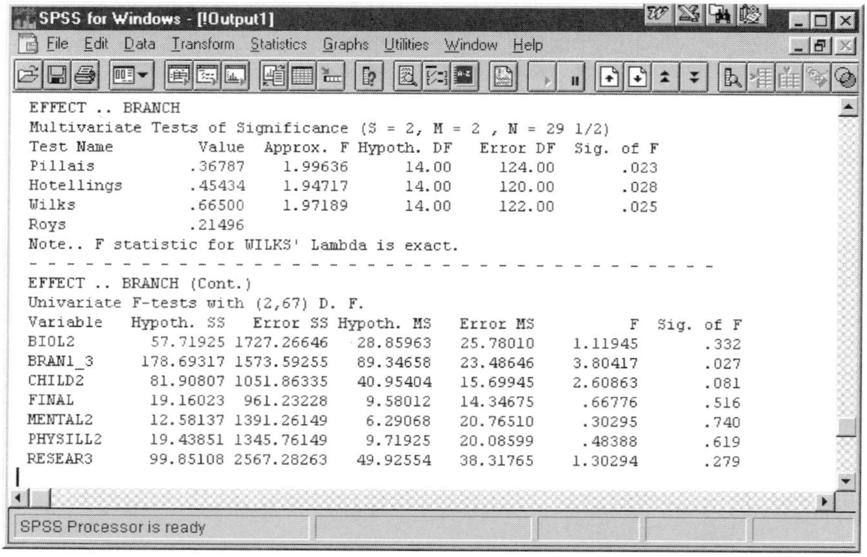

Figure 6.8 MANOVA (seven variables): SPSS Output screen.

health course sat by all students in year two before they opt for a particular branch. We might expect a branch difference here, as those who elect to study child health may be more committed to this area of study. However, we are not permitted to assume that there is a significant difference in this score at an α level of 0.05. None of the other marks is significant, including the final degree mark. This is of practical interest, as it shows that, despite the difference between branches, when all the marks are combined overall no real difference is seen. This is probably because the weightings applied to the courses in the second and third years are much lower than those applied in the fourth year, where no differences are noted among the branches, and also because of the large number of courses (not all shown here) where no differences are seen. Here we see that the statistical significance of a result does not necessarily result in a meaningful or practical difference.

The data being examined here comes from three course branches, but also from different years (1991 to 1994). Any differences could be due to year, branch, or some combination of these two factors. Suppose it were thought that the poorer performance of the child health branch was really due to a particularly bad cohort of students, rather than a general branch effect. What if it is thought that some more complicated relationship exists; perhaps the effect of being in a given year *and* in a given branch combine in some way to give a student a better or worse mark.

TWO-WAY ANOVA

More complicated relationships can be examined using ANOVA models. One-way ANOVA is really a special case of an ANOVA model, with one independent variable and one dependent variable. However, we can have two independent variables, i.e. the variability of the data is explained by two factors. This is called two-way ANOVA. We can also add in interactions between the two independent variables. In the following analysis we will look at the effect of year and branch, both separately and as an interaction.

The SPSS Output screen shown in Figure 6.9 was obtained by selecting the Simple Factorial option of ANOVA Models and using Year and Branch as factors and BRAN1_3 as the dependent variable. The analysis attempts to allocate variance to factors and combinations of factors. The effect of year combined with branch is not found to be significant, nor is the effect of year, but that of branch is significant ($p = 0.015$). The analysis has calculated that a proportion of the variance is explained by these factors, while the remainder of the variance (the *residual variance*) is assumed to be due to random factors.

SPSS allows the analysis of many factors and up to five-way interactions among them, although it is most unlikely you will ever need to use this level of complexity.

SPSS for Windows - [!Output1]

File Edit Data Transform Statistics Graphs Utilities Window Help

```
* * * A N A L Y S I S   O F   V A R I A N C E * * *
          BRAN1_3  Branch Specific M15/Well chil/
      by  BRANCH   Branch (Adult, Child or Mental Health)
          YEAR
          UNIQUE sums of squares
          All effects entered simultaneously
```

Source of Variation	Sum of Squares	DF	Mean Square	F	Sig of F
Main Effects	269.074	4	67.269	2.881	.027
BRANCH	206.707	2	103.353	4.427	.015
YEAR	34.410	2	17.205	.737	.481
2-Way Interactions	138.986	4	34.747	1.488	.212
BRANCH YEAR	138.986	4	34.747	1.488	.212
Explained	553.827	8	69.228	2.965	.005
Residual	2147.980	92	23.348		
Total	2701.807	100	27.018		

SPSS Processor is ready

Figure 6.9 Two-way ANOVA: SPSS Output screen.

REPEATED-MEASURES ANOVA

One of the conditions of ANOVA is that the data are independent, i.e. the same condition applies as for Student's *t*-test (which is a special case of ANOVA, as noted above). However, sometimes we want to look at related measures. We know that a special form of Student's *t*-test, the related or paired *t*-test, addresses this problem, and in ANOVA there is also a special form that deals with more than two related measures. This form of ANOVA may be considered an extension of the related *t*-test to more than two measures.

Carrying on with our examination example, what if the branch coordinators wanted to know if their students had significantly different overall examination marks in years two, three and four? We cannot use ANOVA as the same students are being examined each year, so the data are not independent. In this case we use repeated-measures ANOVA, which is available under ANOVA Models in SPSS.

Repeated measures can become very complex in design, but the present example is fairly straightforward. We need at least one Within Subject factor, which comprises the variables we are repeating for a given subject. Here the factor is the end of year marks, and there are three of them (called year1, year2 and year3 in our SPSS database). Thus the number of levels that SPSS will request we enter is three. We next need to define what the three levels are, and clicking on Define allows us to specify the variables at each of the three levels. Finally, we enter the Between Subjects factor, which in this case could again be Branch, and again we need to define the range of values Branch takes. If we left out the Between Subjects factor we would get simply a measure of whether students in general had significantly different marks across years. The initial steps for stating the level of factors are shown in Figure 6.10. Having entered a factor name (it

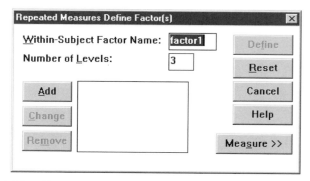

Figure 6.10   Adding Within Subject factors in repeated measures ANOVA: SPSS dialogue box.

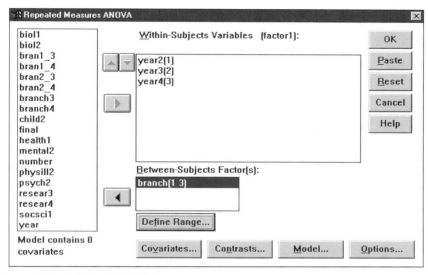

Figure 6.11 Defining Within Subject and between subject factors in repeated-measures ANOVA: SPSS dialogue box.

does not matter what it is called, by default it will be factor1) and the number of levels, we click on Add, which will have the effect of making the Define button selectable. Once we click on Define we get the dialogue box shown in Figure 6.11, where we have filled in the three variables and Between Subjects factor.

We then obtain the Output window shown in Figure 6.12. It can be seen that any difference between years is unlikely to be due to branch differences ($p = 0.36$) but that there is a significant difference in marks from year to year. In fact the means (not shown above) are higher in year four than in the other two years, and year two scores higher than year three. This could be explained by students working hardest at the end of the degree (although we have no proof for this).

WHEN ANOVA IS NOT APPROPRIATE

If data are not normally distributed then we cannot use parametric tests, and ANOVA is a parametric test. A non-parametric alternative to one-way ANOVA is the Kruskal–Wallis test, which does a similar job of comparing more than two groups of (typically ordinal) non-normal data. More than two related variables can be tested to see if they come from the same population by using Friedman's test; this is similar to repeated-measures ANOVA.

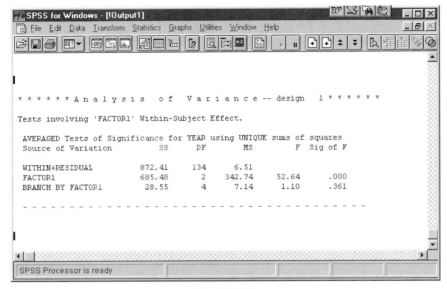

Figure 6.12   Repeated-measures ANOVA: SPSS Output screen.

However, the flexibility to explore complex experimental designs and the power of ANOVA is such that if you can you should transform your data so that they are normally distributed (often this is done by using a log transform). SPSS has a Transform option that allows you to create a new variable by transforming a pre-existing one.

EXERCISES

1. Using infant mortality data, the output shown below was obtained with a one-way ANOVA design, with infant mortality as the dependent variable, and type of country as the independent (grouping) variable. Group 1 is countries of central and eastern Europe, group 2 is European Union countries and group 3 is countries formerly of the USSR. Would you say that the result was sigificant? Interpret the meaning of the output.

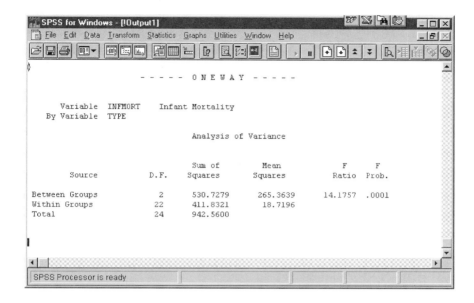

2. A Scheffé's test was computed using the group means shown in the output below. What do the results tell you about the group differences (if any).

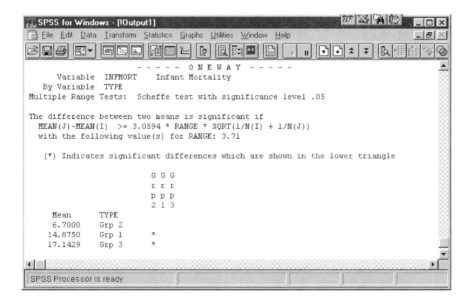

3. To assess the statement that any differences in infant mortality are merely due to economic situations, an ANOVA was done using GNP (gross national

product) as a covariate. The results are given below. Does GNP really explain the change in infant mortality, or is there some effect over and above GNP?

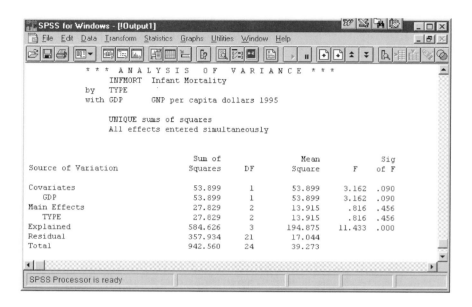

```
SPSS for Windows - [!Output1]
 File  Edit  Data  Transform  Statistics  Graphs  Utilities  Window  Help

        * * *  A N A L Y S I S   O F   V A R I A N C E  * * *
            INFMORT   Infant Mortality
        by   TYPE
        with GDP        GNP per capita dollars 1995

            UNIQUE sums of squares
            All effects entered simultaneously

                                Sum of                    Mean              Sig
    Source of Variation         Squares     DF          Square       F      of F

    Covariates                  53.899       1          53.899    3.162     .090
        GDP                     53.899       1          53.899    3.162     .090
    Main Effects                27.829       2          13.915     .816     .456
        TYPE                    27.829       2          13.915     .816     .456
    Explained                  584.626       3         194.875   11.433     .000
    Residual                   357.934      21          17.044
    Total                      942.560      24          39.273

SPSS Processor is ready
```

REFERENCES

1. Hand D J, Taylor C C 1987 Multivariate analysis of variance and repeated measures. Chapman & Hall, London
2. Naughten V 1998 An exploration of differences in branch marks in a nursing degree programme. BNURS Thesis, School of Health (Nursing), University of Birmingham, UK
3. Glantz S A 1980 Biostatistics: How to detect, correct and prevent errors in medical literature. Circulation 61 (1): 1–7
4. MacArthur R D, Jackson G G 1984 An evaluation of the use of statistical methods in the *Journal of Infectious Diseases*. Journal of Infectious Diseases 149 (3): 349–354

Regression

This chapter discusses a common statistical technique, regression analysis, which explores the possible relationship between two or more variables. It starts with the most common technique, simple linear regression, which attempts to predict one (dependent) variable from another (independent) variable. More complex regression models include multiple regression (several independent variables) and logistic regression (where the dependent variable is binary), which are also considered.

KEY POINTS

- Regression is based on correlation
- A regression analysis assumes linearity
- Regression gives the formula for a linear relationship between two or more variables
- Regression may be used to predict one variable from another
- Logistic regression may be used on a binary dependent variable, and gives the probability of the variable having a given value

At the end of this chapter the student should be able to:

1. State the conditions of regression analysis

2. Set up SPSS for linear regression, multiple regression and logistic regression

101

3. Interpret the results from the SPSS output for linear regression, multiple regression and logistic regression.

INTRODUCTION

Simple linear regression explores possible relationships among data of a linear nature, i.e. where the relationship can be modelled as a straight line. As an example of a linear relationship consider Figure 7.1, which shows a plot of inches against centimetres. For any value in inches, you can read off the corresponding value in centimetres, and vice versa. You can see that 10 inches (inches are on the x axis) corresponds to about 25 centimetres (on the y axis). In fact we do not even need the graph, as the following formula gives the exact relationship:

Centimetres $= 2.54 \times$ inches

Note the following aspects of this graph:

- The relationship is exact, if you know the value in inches then you know the precise value in centimetres
- Zero inches is also zero centimetres, so the line goes through the origin of the graph ($x = 0$, $y = 0$)
- The relationship is a straight line, another word for this is *linear*
- The relationship is positive, i.e. as the number of inches increases so does the number of centimetres.

It is possible to construct relationships that obey none of the above. For

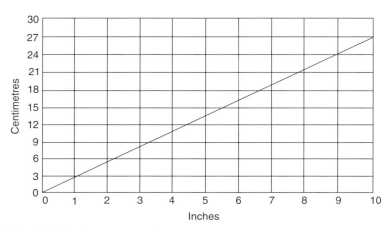

Figure 7.1 Plot of inches versus centimetres.

example, consider the relationship between the dose of a drug that slows the heart beat and pulse rate:

- The relationship is not exact, you cannot predict with certainty that a given dose will result in a particular pulse rate. This is because a patient's pulse depends on other factors (exercise, stress, time of day, etc.). However, the drug does, on average, exert a measurable effect; it is simply that we cannot be absolutely sure of its precise effect.
- If no drug is given the heart still beats, so if the relationship could be modelled as a straight line it would not go through the origin, as zero drug is not associated with zero heart beat (fortunately).
- The relationship need not be linear, and definitely will not be outside a certain range. For if the dose takes the heart beat too low the patient may die, resulting in a pulse rate of zero, but a still higher dose cannot give a lower pulse rate.
- If the drug dose is increased the heart beat slows down more. The relationship is negative.

The relationship is shown graphically in Figure 7.2. Note that three of the above features are evident by inspection:

- The relationship is not exact. While there is an overall trend observable (as the drug dose is increased the heart rate decreases (shown by the straight line)), the actual drug dose and pulse values (the small squares) do not lie on the line, but are scattered around it.

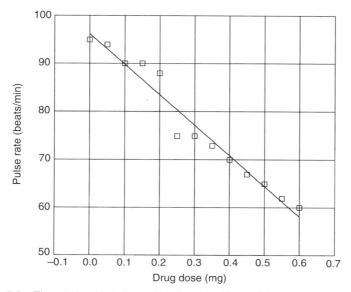

Figure 7.2 The relationship between the dose of a (fictional) heart drug and pulse rate.

- The line that best fits the relationship (the straight line) does not go through the origin.
- The slope of the line is negative, i.e. as the dose is increased the pulse rate decreases.

You will probably recognize the graph in Figure 7.2 as a scatterplot. It shows that the two variables are correlated. Regression is based on correlation, and uses the correlation coefficient to produce the straight line that gives the best guess of what one variable will be, given the value of the other. For example, if no drug is given we would expect the heart rate to be 96 beats/min; in fact we record it was 95. We would guess that a dose of 0.4 mg would result in a heart rate of about 70 beats/min, but we may record a different pulse rate. However, it is clear that 70 beats/min would be a better estimate than (say) 110 beats/min, as none of the patients with such high pulses are receiving doses as high as 0.4 mg: the three patients with a pulse rate of 100–110 beats/min are receiving doses of 0.05–0.15 mg, whereas patients with a pulse rate of 60–70 beats/min are receiving doses above 0.3 mg. Therefore, while the prediction is inexact, it is still helpful.

LINEAR REGRESSION

In the above examples you may have wondered how we decided where to draw the straight line through the points. You may also wonder whether it is even appropriate to draw such a line, in other words are we deluding ourselves that there is a relationship between the drug dose and pulse rate? It is the technique of linear regression that answers both these questions. For further texts on regression, especially with respect to the relevant software packages, see references 1–5.

Linear regression has three main outputs:

- The probability that a straight line describes the relationship between the two variables
- The slope of the line
- The point where the line crosses the x axis.

If you know where the line crosses the x axis, and how steep (the *slope*) the line is, you can draw the line. There is a very simple equation that defines any straight line:

$$y = (\text{Slope} \times x) + \text{Constant}$$

where the constant is the value of y at which the line crosses the y axis (i.e. the value of y when $x = 0$); this is also called the *intercept*. You will often see this equation written as

$$y = mx + c,$$

where c is the constant and m is the slope.

In the inches and centimetres example (Fig. 7.1), the equation is

$$\text{Centimetres} = 2.54 \times \text{Inches} + 0$$

i.e. the slope of the line is 2.54, and the constant is zero. While you may find reading the value off the graph easier than working it out from the formula, in fact the equation and the graph are identical in the information they contain.

Conditions

Regression makes the following requirements of the data:

- *Normality*. Regression is a parametric test, and assumes that the data are normally distributed.
- *Linearity*. A linear relation exists between the dependent and independent variables. Thus it is sensible to model the relationship as a straight line.
- *Independence*. The data should have been drawn independently. In the drug dose versus pulse rate example above, several pulse readings from the same person should not have been used.
- *Unexplained variance*. The portion of the variance of the dependent variable not explained by the independent variable is due to random error and follows a normal distribution (a normal distribution is one that has a bell-shaped curve, most values lie in in the middle (close to the mean), and as one moves away from the central values, the number of subjects drops off in number). The regression module in SPSS allows the option of saving the residuals (the difference between the predicted values according to the regression equation and the actual values). These residuals can be checked for normality using the Kolmogorov–Smirnov test (for example) or can be shown as a histogram. Figure 7.3 shows such a histogram, which is not obviously normal, although in this case the Kolmogorov–Smirnov test indicates that the data could be normal ($p = 0.925$). The data should not exhibit heteroscedasticity, where the scatter around the line of best fit varies a lot as one proceeds along the line. Figure 7.2 shows no apparent change in scatter as you move along the best fit, and thus shows little or no heteroscedasticity.

Example: Examination marks

Suppose we wished to predict those students who are likely to do well in the

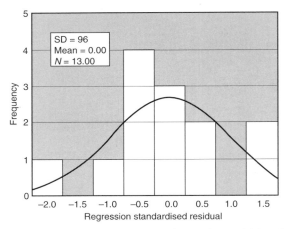

Figure 7.3   The residuals of a regression equation (dependent variable pulse rate).

dissertation in the final year of nursing degree. We could suppose that, as the dissertation requires the student to use the skills studied in the research course, the best predictor would be how well the student did in the research coursework and examination, which was held in the third year.

Figure 7.4 shows a scatterplot of the mark obtained for the dissertation against the research course mark. Despite a large variation between the two marks, it looks as though higher marks in the dissertation do, on average, correspond to higher research course marks. A Pearson correlation coefficient, obtained in SPSS by selecting Statistics then Correlate then Bivariate, and putting the two variables RESEAR3 and RESEAR4 as variables, give the output shown in Figure 7.5.

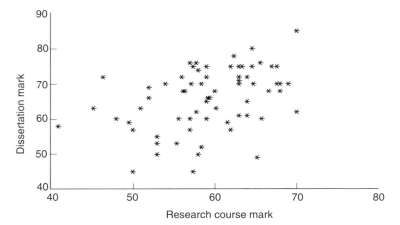

Figure 7.4   Plot of the mark obtained for the research dissertation against the mark obtained in the research course examination (both as marks out of 100).

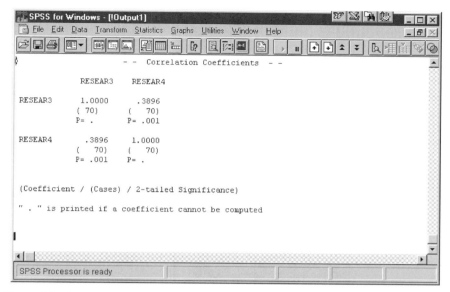

Figure 7.5 Pearson correlation coefficients: SPSS Output screen.

In SPSS all variables are correlated with each other variable selected. Here, there are only two variables, so only one useful correlation is produced (the correlation of RESEAR3 with itself is clearly unity, and of no interest, as is the correlation of RESEAR4 with itself; and the correlation of RESEAR4 with RESEAR3 is identical with the correlation of RESEAR3 with RESEAR4). A correlation of about 0.4 is found, which is a moderate correlation, but it is highly significant ($p = 0.001$).

So we can see that as the mark for RESEAR3 increases so does that for RESEAR4. In other words the previous work of the students gives a rough guide of how well they will do in the dissertation, but because other factors are also relevant it is not sensible to think we can exactly predict one mark from the last. Other factors that may affect the mark gained in the dissertation are, for example, a student may work extra hard because of a previous bad mark, another student may fall ill or be under extra stress before the dissertation and not work as effectively, and a different examiner (or even the same one) may mark work of a similar standard differently.

What we would like to do is to create a graph similar to the one in Figure 7.2 but that shows us the relationship between RESEAR3 and RESEAR4. We want to be able to produce a best guess for RESEAR4 based on the RESEAR3 mark, although clearly we cannot predict RESEAR4 with absolute certainty.

Regression is the technique that will give us this relationship. It will furnish us with a straight line that best fits the data. As shown above, the straight line can be completely described by two values: the slope and the constant (the intercept). SPSS calls the constant the value B in the Constant row, and the slope is the value B in the Variable row (here RESEAR3). The reasons for this apparently clumsy notation will become clearer later.

Regression assumes that there is at least one independent variable and one dependent variable, where the dependent variable is being predicted from the independent variable. In this case it is clearly more sensible to predict year 4 results from year 3 results rather than the other way around.

Linear regression is obtained in SPSS by selecting Statistics, then Regression, then Linear. Putting the variable RESEAR4 into dependent variable and RESEAR3 into independent variables in the resulting dialogue box, and leaving all other options as the default, gives the output shown in Figure 7.6. The output looks complex, but we can break it down into simpler components.

First, SPSS reports some general information, with the default settings for the regression analysis, which need not concern us yet. Next, it states which variable (RESEAR4) is being predicted, this is the dependent variable (because it depends on the value of some other variable(s)), and which variable is being used to make the prediction (RESEAR3), this is the independent variable (because this does not depend on any other variable, but is given, and is being used to predict RESEAR4). Note that, while we are

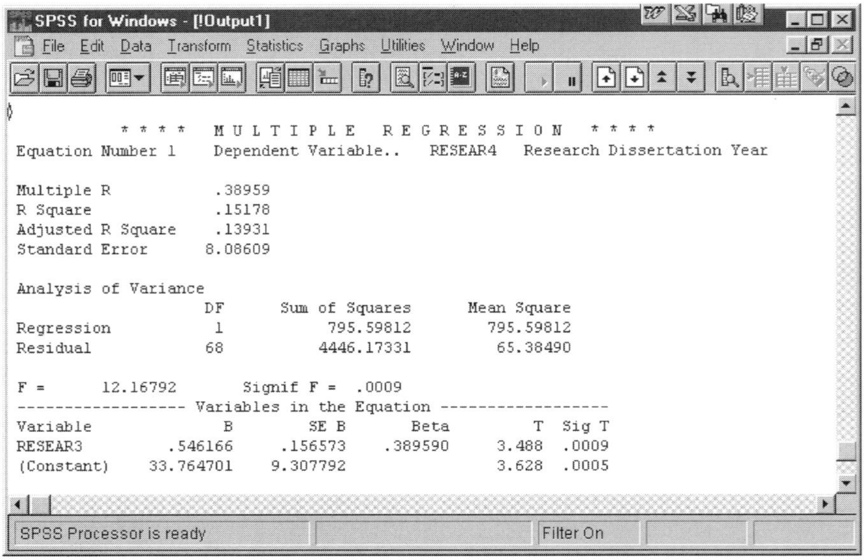

Figure 7.6   Linear regression: SPSS Output screen.

using simple linear regression here, SPSS considers this as a particularly simple case of multiple regression.

SPSS then reports the Multiple R, which is identical to the correlation coefficient between RESEAR3 and RESEAR4. This is not coincidental, as regression starts with the correlation coefficient. The square of R is useful as it can be shown that this gives the percentage of the variance of the data that is explained by the regression. In the present case, 15.178% of the variance in RESEAR4 is explained by RESEAR3; the remaining variance is due to other factors. Thus, while RESEAR3 may be a useful predictor, most of the mark in RESEAR4 is not purely due to the RESEAR3 mark; in fact about 85% seems to be due to other factors. SPSS also gives a value called the Adjusted R Square, which is a more conservative estimate than R^2.

The regression equation is given at the bottom of the box. Here we are only interested in predicting RESEAR4 from one other variable (RESEAR3), but more complex regression, called multiple regression (see below), can be achieved, so in general more than one variable might be reported. The value of the slope of the line is shown as B in the RESEAR3 line (here about 0.55). The other values shown on the line for RESEAR3 are shown again below:

Variable	B	SE B	Beta	T	Sig T
RESEAR3	0.546 166	0.156 573	0.389 590	3.488	0.000 9

The value of B is not known with precision, and the standard error is quoted as about 0.16. A significance based on a T statistic is given as $p < 0.001$ (actual value 0.0009), so we are very confident that the relationship is significant.

A similar analysis is done on the constant:

Variable	B	SE B	Beta	T	Sig T
(Constant)	33.764 701	9.307 792		3.628	0.000 5

The value of the constant is also shown as B, though in this case in the (Constant) line, and is about 33.8. This value is also tested for significance, and is also found to be very significant ($p = 0.0005$).

The regression equation can now be stated as

RESEAR4 = 0.55 × RESEAR3 + 33.8

So if a student had a RESEAR3 mark of 50, my best guess for RESEAR4 would be

RESEAR4 = 0.55 × 50 + 33.8 = 61.3

Note this implies that, on average, students do better in RESEAR4 than RESEAR3.

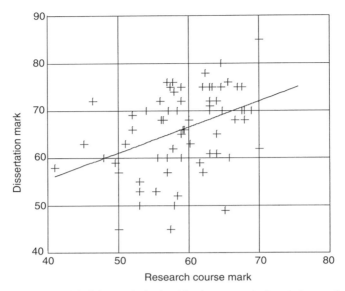

Figure 7.7 Linear model of the mark obtained for the research dissertation against the mark obtained in the research course examination (both as marks out of 100).

Another way of visualizing this relation is shown in Figure 7.7. This plot was obtained in SPSS by selecting Statistics, then Regression, then Curve Estimation, and then putting the same variables in dependent and independent variables. This procedure allows you to try to fit many different relationships to the data, but the default is linear. If you click on the Edit button in the resultant graph that appears in the SPSS chart carousel, you can change the appearance of the graph. I have changed Figure 7.7 to show the marks as separate crosses by selecting Attributes, then Interpolation, then None, as by default the chart shows all the points joined up as a line. I have also added a grid and made a few other minor edits.

Figure 7.7 shows the actual points, and the best fit line, which is the *regression line*. We can see that a mark of 50 on RESEAR3 does indeed correspond to a mark of just over 60 in RESEAR4.

MULTIPLE REGRESSION

We have seen that, while the RESEAR4 mark can to some extent be predicted from RESEAR3, most of the variability (85%) results from other factors about the student. Possibly the skills assessed by RESEAR3 are only part of the factors that explain a student's performance in the dissertation. RESEAR3 is largely theoretical statistics and methodology; other courses cover clinical areas that might be very useful in devising and

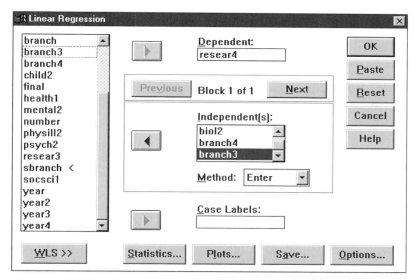

Figure 7.8   Linear regression: SPSS dialogue box.

writing up a real-life project. We can explore these additional courses as possible factors by using multiple regression. Using the same menu selection as for simple linear regression, but adding in several other variables, can be achieved via the dialogue box shown in Figure 7.8, where some of the independent variables have been entered. Note that, by default, the Method is set to Enter, which means that all variables are used in the regression, even if they are found not to be significant. There are several options for only keeping those variables that are found to be significant, and I opted to change the Method to Step before executing this analysis. Stepwise regression adds or removes variables from the analysis, depending on the Options selected. By default, a variable is entered if $p < 0.05$, and removed if $p > 0.1$.

The output (Fig. 7.9) is similar to that for simple linear regression, but the dependent variable is now assumed to be predictable from more than one independent variable. The output shows that in fact only RESEAR3 seems to be relevant in this analysis; knowing the other marks does not seem to help, as all the other variables have significances above the α level (called Criterion PIN, and here put at 0.05; not shown in Fig. 7.9). The interpretation is that of the data collected, only RESEAR3 seems to help predict the dissertation mark.

However, the same may not be true of other marks. Consider the BRANCH4 mark, this is the combined coursework and examination mark for branch-specific work. We might presume that this should be related to

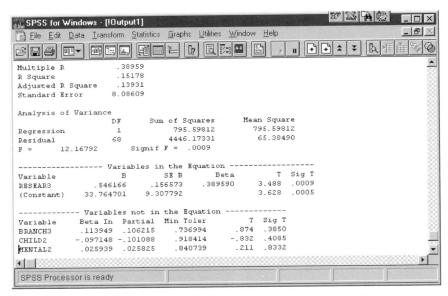

Figure 7.9   Multiple regression: SPSS Output screen (only part of full SPSS window is shown in this screen).

the branch-specific mark for year 3, BRANCH3, but are there any other marks that could help predict this mark? Look at the output box shown in Figure 7.10. Here BRANCH4 is the dependent variable and the other courses are independent variables. The output was obtained with SPSS, using the same options as before. The analysis proceeds through several iterations, adding and removing variables until it cannot remove or add according to the criteria we set in the Options dialogue box.

Note that here SPSS has kept two of the variables, BRANCH3 and PHYSILL2. Thus, while (unsurprisingly) the branch programme in year three is a good predictor, the branch-specific course can be predicted with greater accuracy by adding PHYSILL2 to the equation. We can now explain one of the other aspects of regression, the Beta value. This gives a measure of how important each variable is, in a normalized range of zero to one, and we see here that PHYSILL2 seems to be the more important of the two variables in predicting the year 4 branch marks.

For multiple regression, the equation $y = mx + c$, which in SPSS could be stated as

Dependent variable = Independent variable $\times$ B value of independent variable + B value of constant

or, more succinctly,

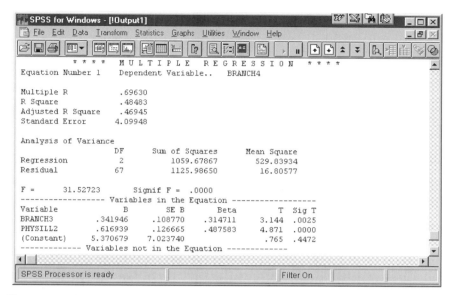

Figure 7.10 Multiple regression: SPSS Output screen (only part of full SPSS window is shown in this screen).

Dependent variable $= B_{var1} \, Var_1 + B_{constant}$

is expanded to (for N independent variables, Var1, Var2, Var3, ..., VarN)

$$\text{Dependent variable} = B_{var1} \, Var1 + B_{var2} \, Var2 + B_{var3} \, Var3 \dots$$
$$+ B_{varN} \, VarN + B_{constant}$$

In the present case we have two significant variables, so

Dependent variable $= B_{var1} \, Var_1 + B_{var2} Var_2 + B_{constant}$

and if we put the values in we get

BRANCH4 = (BRANCH3 × 0.34) + (PHYSILL2 × 0.62) + 5.4

However, as the constant term is not significant ($p = 0.4472$) we might choose to ignore it, and thus we have

BRANCH4 = (BRANCH3 × 0.34) + (PHYSILL2 × 0.62)

So a student who scored 40 on BRANCH3 but 80 on PHYSILL2 would be predicted to score

BRANCH4 = $(40 \times 0.34) + (80 \times 0.62) = 13.6 + 49.6 = 63.5$

If we also include the constant term we obtain a value of about 69. In either case the mark is nearer that of PHYSILL2 than that of BRANCH3 as predicted by the Beta value.

LIMITATIONS TO REGRESSION

Regression is a powerful technique for prediction. There are, however, some limitations to the technique:

• The prediction based on linear regression is not necessarily correct, or even guaranteed to be close. It is simply the best guess on the information available.

• The fact that two or more variables are correlated does not necessarily imply causation. You should have a theoretical rationale for how one variable might predict another before using regression to calculate a predicted value.

• The regression equation may fail outside of the range of values from which it was constructed. For example, based on the regression analysis of for the heart drug where the values of the dose ranged from 0 to 0.5 mg, a very high drug dose of (say) 5 mg may not produce 10 times the reduction in pulse over the pulse that a dose of 0.5 mg produces.

LOGISTIC REGRESSION

Sometimes what we wish to predict is the occurrence or non-occurrence of some event. Certain types of patients suffer from pressure sores much more than other groups (e.g. those with poor nutrition). However we cannot do a regression for nutritional status (as measured by serum albumin, for example) against pressure sore, because a patient can have a sore or not, but cannot have 0.5 of a sore. In other words, the presence or absence of a sore is nominal data and thus cannot be normally distributed (this concept being meaningless for nominal data). Therefore, as it stands, regression is inappropriate.

There is a form of regression, called logistic regression, that can be used where the dependent variable is dichotomous, i.e. can take two values. In the pressure sore case, a sore can exist (we could label this 1) or not exist (we could label this 0). Logistic regression returns a probability, in this case of whether the sore will occur or not.

To perform a logistic regression analysis in SPSS, select Statistics, then Regression, and then Logistic. In a study conducted in the West Midlands, wheelchair patients were assessed using the Waterlow score,[6] a scale developed for elderly hospital patients. The score consists of several subscores that assess features known to be associated with sore formation. It is of interest to know whether this score works on wheelchair patients, and if so which portions of it are useful.

In the study patients were assessed using the Waterlow score, and were also assessed to see if a sore was present. One of the parameters of the Waterlow score is the state of the skin, which would give a high score if reddened (for example) or if a sore was already present. Consequently, unless we do a predictive study (i.e. following up patients who initially did not have a sore), it is not useful to analyse this particular variable, and thus it was excluded from the analysis. While one could argue that the presence of a sore could affect some of the variables (e.g. mobility – if you have a sore you may be less likely to be mobile), it was considered useful to explore them in this convenience study, if only to look at whether they might be useful in a later study. Other factors, such as gender, can clearly not be affected by whether the patient has a sore or not.

The subscores looked at were:

WTRAUMA	Recent injury/surgery, etc.
WMOBIL	Mobility
WSEX	Gender
WAGE	Age
WAPPET	Appetite
WBUILD	Body build
WCONT	Continence
WMEDIC	Medication
WNEURO	Neurological deficit
WSPECIAL	Other special risk factors (e.g. smoking)

The SPSS output of the analysis is shown in Figure 7.11. The salient features of the output are described below.

A total of 150 subjects were analysed. Since none of them had a score for WTRAUMA, it was constant (0) for all of them, and was therefore useless as a predictor (it would always say the same thing) and has been excluded by SPSS. Logistic regression, like multiple regression, allows variables to be excluded or included according to various algorithms and options. I used the Forward Wald method, which starts off with no variables, and adds variables if they are significant, stopping when no more significant ones are found.

An equation has been constructed using those variables found to be significant which computes the likelihood of getting a sore for given values of the significant variables. The formula is then used to classify the subjects into those with and those without sores. Patients were considered to be in the predicted sore group if the value of the predicted probability was greater than 0.5, and were considered to be in the predicted non-sore

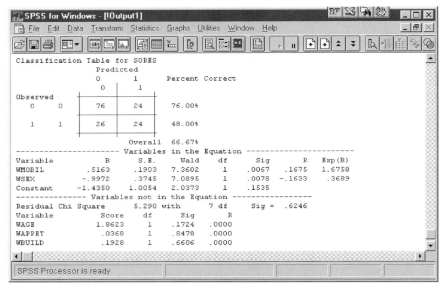

Figure 7.11 Logistic regression: SPSS Output screen (only part of full SPSS window is shown in this screen).

group otherwise. These predictions are compared to whether the patients actually had a sore, and the correct percentage is given. Here we see that nearly half (48%) of those who had a sore were identified as having one, and over three-quarters (76%) of those that did not have a sore were correctly identified.

The variables found significant are then given, and we see that only two were found to be useful: mobility and gender. None of the other variables were used in the classification. In the Waterlow score a higher score is assigned to female than male, but the analysis here gives a negative sign for this variable, indicating that it works in the opposite direction (i.e. it is men who are more at risk). So, we can see that in a new score for wheelchair patients, the score for gender should be reversed.

I should point out that the study is very much a pilot study, and the above analysis is not definitive. However, it has been used to plan a new prospective and much larger study (funded by the Smith & Nephew Foundation), which I will complete about the time this book goes on sale.

Logistic regression in SPSS allows you to save various results, including the probability of getting (in this case) a sore. You can use this to store results for receiver operating characteristic (ROC) analysis (see Ch. 8).

CONCLUSION

Regression is a technique for predicting one dependent variable from one (simple linear regression) or more (multiple regression) independent variables. It makes assumptions about the data (e.g. normality and linearity), and the results may be nonsensical if there is no clear reason why a causal relationship should exist. If the dependent variable is binary (e.g. yes/no, on/off, male/female) then logistic regression may be employed to determine the probability of one or other value of the variable being obtained.

EXERCISES

Using the data in the Output window shown below, where the variables WATMOBIL, WATAGE and WATBUILD are the Waterlow components for mobility, age and build, respectively, answer the following questions:

1. Which of the variables WATAGE and WATBUILD, if either, appears to be useful in predicting WATMOBIL?

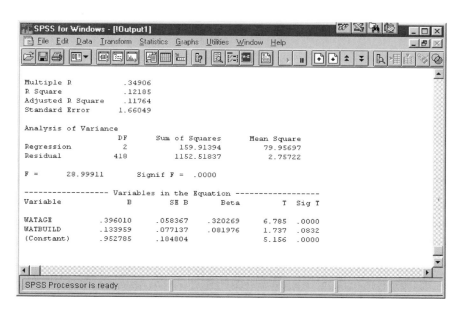

2. Write down the formula for predicting WATMOBIL.

3. What percentage of the variance of WATMOBIL is accounted for by the regression equation where both variables and the constant are used?

4. This regression was computed using the method Enter, what might have been a more useful method?

REFERENCES

1. Abacus Concepts 1992 Statview. Abacus Concepts, Berkeley, C A, p 300–319
2. Chatfield C 1978 Statistics for technology. Chapman & Hall, London, p 166–202
3. Hammond S 1995 Introduction to multivariate data analysis. In: Brakwell G M, Hammond S, Fife-Schaw C (eds) Research methods in psychology. Sage, London, p 360–385
4. Norusis M J 1993 SPSS for Windows base system user's guide. SPSS, Chicago, IL
5. Ryan B F, Joiner B L, Ryan T A 1995 Minitab. Duxbury Press, Boston, MA, p 218–259
6. Waterlow J 1995 A risk assessment card. Nursing Times 27(49): 51–55

8

Receiver operating characteristic (ROC)

This chapter discusses the receiver operating characteristic (ROC), which is a technique used in classification analysis. ROC analysis is well known in psychology, medicine, medical physics, chemistry and medical imaging, but is not well known in many branches of health care. For a good introduction to its use in psychology see Rose[1] and for medical imaging see Swets.[2] A summary for medicine is given in Altman & Bland[3,4] and a detailed description can be found in Zweig & Campbell.[5]

KEY POINTS

- Sensitivity is a measure of detection of abnormal cases
- Specificity measures the detection of normal cases
- For a given risk assessment scale, specificity is inversely related to sensitivity
- Both sensitivity and specificity are used in ROC
- The area under a ROC curve can be used to directly compare the classification by two or more scales, techniques, human assessors, etc.

At the end of this chapter the student should be able to:

1. Calculate sensitivity and specificity

2. Plot a ROC curve

3. Compare two assessment methods using ROC

INTRODUCTION

The accuracy of diagnosis of distal fractures and the prediction of pressure sores show the worth of ROC in areas such as nursing or physiotherapy. The excellent STEPS software, a component of the Teaching and Learning Technology Programme (TLTP) programme for computer-based learning, available to bona fide academics and students free of charge, has a thorough CBL package devoted to ROC.[6] (The STEPS software also contains many other components addressing examples in various disciplines. While these do not include health care, the psychology and biology sections have many examples highly relevant to health care and medicine. The software is not highly dependent on any particular package, although Minitab is assumed in some cases to be the package in use. The URL for the TLTP program is available at http://www.tltp.ac.uk, and much of the software can be down-loaded from this site.)

The potential use for ROC will be any area where decisions are made, where you are not certain when you are right, and where the decisions can be made with various levels of confidence. This is typical of most health care decisions, and all of the interesting ones (i.e. the decisions that require some expertise). ROC has been little used in some areas of health care – nursing and physiotherapy, for example. In a review of nursing research textbooks and statistics texts aimed at nurses, no mention of ROC has been found by me. In a review of all articles published in the whole of 1984 and the last six months of 1994 in the *Journal of Advanced Nursing*[7] I found no study that used ROC.

Diagnosis of fractures is a new area for nursing, and is part of the advanced practitioner role for nurses in some accident and emergency departments. Classification involves placing objects that are similar to each other (e.g. diseases) into a group. A person with a given set of signs and symptoms is given a specific diagnosis. In the example given in this chapter, radiographs are used to split those who have a fracture from those who do not.

But how accurate are nurses at diagnosing fractures? Diagnosis from a radiograph can be complex, and you can make a mistake. The nurse can be perfect at picking up fractures by always saying that there is a fracture, as then she will miss none, but nor will she ever declare a radiograph clear. The technical description of such a classification is that it is very *sensitive*, in that no fracture is missed; but it is not *specific* at all, in that all radiographs are said to show a fracture. These two terms will be discussed and defined below, but sensitivity measures how good we are at picking up the disease, and specificity how good we are at identifying the normal. The above is clearly a very extreme case, but shows that a very sensitive measure is not necessarily useful. At the other extreme a nurse may never say a radiograph shows a fracture, and by missing all fractures that do occur shows a low sensitivity (in fact zero). However, she does not ever mis-interpret a normal radiograph as showing a fracture, and is said to have a high specificity. Clearly this form of classification is useless also. Thus ensuring that you never make a mistake in misinterpreting a fracture as normal, or never making the opposite mistake of misinterpreting a normal radiograph as showing a fracture will not typically give a useful classification.

By looking at the sensitivity and the specificity of the diagnosis together, ROC can assess the nurse and compare her ability with other professionals. This will clearly be necessary if nurses are to be accepted as 'safe' in this new domain for nursing practice. Overton[8] used ROC to compare nurses with casualty officers with regard to the assessment of distal fractures, and found no significant differences between the two groups. This study gives quantitative evidence that nurses are competent in this new area.

Similarly, you might want to predict those patients who will develop pressure sores by using a system that splits patients who are high risk for developing a pressure sore, according to some scoring system. Again the system is most unlikely to be 100% accurate; many patients stated to be at high risk will not develop sores, and some who at not considered at risk may do so. The concept of a threshold is inherent in such a system, as the patient is given a score indicating risk. But at which score do we consider them at risk? We can choose any score as the one that defines risk, but we will typically want the threshold score to split the patients into those likely to develop sores and those unlikely to develop sores, which is not necessarily (or usually) the same thing as splitting them into those that definitely will not from those that definitely will develop sores. If the score indicates increasing risk, raising the threshold will result in a less sensitive tool, and lowering the threshold will give a more sensitive one. Unfortunately, as shown above, the more sensitive measure is not necessarily a better one.

SENSITIVITY AND SPECIFICITY

Let us now define these two concepts. When making a binary decision, as for example deciding on the diagnosis of a fracture or no fracture (it is or it is not a fracture, there are two cases), one may make a true diagnosis where the fracture is present or absent, or a false diagnosis, also where the fracture is present or absent. There are four cases in total:

- *True-positive decision*: the patient has a fracture (disease, will develop a sore etc.) and we state they do
- *True-negative decision*: the patient does not have a fracture etc. and we state this correctly
- *False-positive decision*: the patient does not have a fracture etc. but we state they do
- *False-negative decision*: the patient has a fracture etc., but we say they do not.

True positive and true negative rates can be used together to give measures of accuracy.

Sensitivity is identical to a true positive ratio. It is defined as the proportion of all positive cases that are correctly identified as positive. Sensitivity measures how well we perform in identifying those subjects with a fracture (or other condition). As all the positive cases comprise those that we got right (true positives) and those we got wrong (false negatives), the ratio of true positive to all positives is given by

$$\text{Sensitivity} = \frac{\text{True positive}}{\text{True positive} + \text{False negative}}$$

Specificity is defined as the proportion of all negative cases that are correctly identified as negative. Specificity measures how well we perform in identifying those subjects who are normal (i.e. do not have a fracture or some other condition of interest). As all the negative cases comprise those that we got right (true negative) and those we got wrong (false positive), the ratio of true negative to all negatives is given by

$$\text{Specificity} = \frac{\text{True negative}}{\text{True negative} + \text{False positive}}$$

Specificity is the same as the true negative ratio. In practice the false positive ratio is often used. The true negatives and false positives are all the negative cases, and it follows that the true negative ratio and false positive ratios add to unity. Using the false positive ratio is therefore identical to using (1 – specificity).

Sensitivity and specificity are simply the number of correct cases as a fraction of the totals for those patients who have/do not have the condition.

THRESHOLDS

One does not typically state with absolute certainty that, for example, a patient has a fracture or that a patient will develop a pressure sore, or that they do not have a fracture or will not develop a sore. A more natural statement would be that one is very sure, or fairly confident, or that it is quite unlikely, etc.

However, sometimes a straightforward choice of where to allocate resources requires a decision to be made, even if we cannot be 100% sure of what the right decision is; so we need a best guess. For example, the patient is at high risk of pressure sore formation and therefore needs a special mattress, or they are not and the mattress can be allocated to someone else. Thus one needs to identify a threshold above which the patient is at high risk and below which they are not. For example, the Waterlow score above which a patient is said to be at high risk could be stated to be 10. In this case any value above 10 (the threshold) is said to indicate risk. It is also possible to have a scoring system such as the Braden score, which works in the opposite direction; i.e. low scores are indicative of risk, in which case values below a given threshold would indicate risk.

If it is important to get the diagnosis right and making a false positive diagnosis is not problematic, then one can set the threshold low (or, if increasing score implies less risk, we would set the threshold high, as the scale is the other way round, where decreases in the scale imply more risk). If a patient monitor gives an alarm when there is nothing wrong with the patient, it causes some irritation. However, if the alarm fails to go off and some injury or death could ensue then clearly this is far more important to avoid than the irritation of false alarms. There is a penalty for a false positive alarm, i.e. resetting the alarm, irritation and noise. However, as the penalty for a false negative alarm could be death, we set the monitor to be very sensitive, or to have a low threshold. Thus we accept a poor specificity in this situation in order to ensure a very high sensitivity.

While in health care it is usually important to not miss a true case (a diagnosis of some disease, for example), i.e. a false negative is almost always a problem, sometimes setting an arbitrarily low threshold is not advised. There may be a significant penalty in getting the decision wrong either way; failure to accept true positive, and reject true negative may both be dangerous. For example, if a test shows a patient to have a pulmonary embolism (PE) we would treat with anticoagulants, as PE can be fatal. The penalty for a false-negative diagnosis would therefore be a failure to treat the PE, resulting in death from respiratory arrest. However, unnecessary treatment with anticoagulants can cause dangerous bleeding in post-surgical patients, and therefore a highly sensitive test that always gets the PE cases but also wrongly diagnosis many who do not have the disease could also cause danger. The benefit from a true-positive diagnosis is that the potentially life-threatening condition of PE is treated, and the benefit from a true-negative diagnosis is that iatrogenic bleeding of a patient who does not have PE is prevented.

There is thus a trade-off in setting the threshold level. For example, in mass screening for human immunodeficiency virus (HIV) one might have a blood test where high values indicate a high probability of having the virus and lower values indicate less probability of having the virus. If one sets the threshold too high, many of the population with the condition will not be picked up, while if one sets the threshold too low many of the population will be diagnosed HIV positive who do not in fact have the virus, causing distress.

The level at which one sets the threshold depends on the relative merits of specificity and sensitivity in the given domain. This may be, and often is, a subjective assessment.

CONFIDENCE LEVELS

One method of obtaining several threshold levels simultaneously is to allocate confidence levels to the decisions. For each level of confidence, one measures true positives and false positives as a percentage of the maximum true positives and false positives possible. Thus one could ask clinicians to state how sure, using a score range of 1–5, they were in making a given decision (e.g. a diagnostic decision). Rather than use numerical confidence levels, which could be meaningless to a clinician, the levels could be obtained from a Likert scale, for example a five-point scale such as the one shown below:

5 Very confident that disease is present
4 Quite confident that disease is present
3 Unsure if disease is present or not
2 Quite confident that disease is not present
1 Very confident that disease is not present

In this example, if the level was allocated a number as shown above, then one might set a threshold of 3, whereby any value *more than or equal to* 3 would be considered a positive diagnosis, which would include many cases of 'unsure'. Choosing 4 as the threshold value would remove the 'unsure' cases, with only 'very confident' or 'quite confident' being now considered a positive diagnosis. Thus less false-positive but more false-negative diagnoses would probably ensue.

GOLD STANDARD

If one is to test the classification ability of a person, scoring system, etc., then one needs to know what the correct classification should be. This is not always easy. If one uses a specialist in classifying as the 'gold standard' for determining how well an inexperienced trainee is performing, one implicitly trusts the specialist to always be right – but she may make mistakes. Where possible the 'gold standard' should be objective and demonstrably correct; where this is impossible it should be a classifier that one has much more confidence in than the one being assessed.

In a prospective study the gold standard may be whether the patient ultimately contracts the disease or condition. This may be very clear in some cases (e.g. from post mortem examination).

ASSESSMENT AT MANY DIFFERENT THRESHOLDS: ROC

The sensitivity and specificity is, as shown above, dependent on the threshold used. However, one does not need to insist on using only one threshold. One can use several. ROC is the term applied to the analysis and measurement of sensitivity and specificity at many thresholds simultaneously. The advantage of ROC is that one can decide which threshold is optimal for a given decision-making problem. One can also directly compare different classification systems by looking at the full spectrum of thresholds possible. Without such an approach it is always difficult to compare two systems, as system A may show greater sensitivity than system B simply because it was assessed at a threshold that allowed great sensitivity, while in general system B might actually perform better than system A.

Example: ROC analysis of pressure sore risk

Rather than simply state that a patient will or will not be at risk, a scoring system can be employed. The nurse can decide that anyone over (or under, if low scores indicate high risk) a certain score is at high risk. The score becomes the threshold. However, there are a range of scores to choose from. Which is the best?

The nurse could improve the sensitivity by lowering the threshold at which she decides a sore will form; this will entail less false-negative predictions. However, the number of false-positive predictions is then likely to go up and the specificity will worsen. The threshold therefore has a profound effect on the classification ability. Lower the threshold and sensitivity improves and specificity worsens; raise the threshold and specificity improves and sensitivity worsens. If the scoring system worked in the opposite direction (low scores indicate high risk), then lowering the threshold would have the opposite effect of improving specificity and worsening sensitivity.

Criticisms have been made of the scoring systems used for pressure sores. Cullum et al[9] stated that the scales have been developed ad hoc and no adequate analysis has been made of the systems. It is known that they predict sores in the sense that higher scores (Waterlow) or lower scores (Braden, Norton) are associated with higher sore incidence, but the optimum threshold has not been established. Waterlow, for example, states any patient with a score above 10 is at risk, and higher scores are defined for greater risk,[10] but the basis for selecting these scores is not clear.

In a population of 9022 patients from a district general hospital[11] about 6500 had a score below 10, and none of these patients developed a pressure sore (decubitus ulcer). Of about 1500 patients with a score between 10 and 14 only four developed a pressure sore, and of 842 patients with a score of 15 and above 89 developed sores.

Thus at the threshold suggested by Waterlow (10) all the sores could be predicted, but most of those patients predicted to develop a sore in fact did not do so. Only about 4% of those patients with a score above 10 developed a sore; indeed only about 10% of those with a score of 15 or above developed a sore. Thus the sensitivity at a threshold score of 10 is 100%, while the specificity is about 80%. This seems very satisfactory, as a large number of patients can be excluded from being at risk.

As the threshold score increases the number of patients having scores above the threshold will decrease. This will be true for the patients with sores and those with no sores. However, if the scoring system means anything, we would expect that the higher the score the higher the proportion of sores to non-sores. So what would happen if the scoring system simply does not work? The ratio of patients with sores compared with those with no sores will be the same at each score; or to put it another way, higher scores would not be associated with higher proportions of patients with sores. The ratio of the true positive rate (sensitivity) to the false positive rate (1 – specificity) will therefore be constant. If one plotted a graph of the ratios for each threshold it would give a straight line.

An ROC curve is simply a plot of the true positive rate against the false positive rate for given thresholds. A system that classifies randomly produces a straight line, with the diagonal running from bottom left to top right on the ROC plot.

Going back to our example, only four patients who scored under 15 developed sores, so the York team decided to use 15 as their threshold. Having excluded the subjects scoring under 15, a new analysis was completed. The sensitivity and specificity was measured for each Waterlow score of 15 and above in this reduced dataset. An ROC analysis was produced[12] which showed that focusing on the scores over 15 gave a much better performance than random, thus providing evidence that the Waterlow score does work as a risk indicator. (*Note*: In Anthony[12] the sensitivity and specificity is measured on the reduced dataset after removing all the subjects scoring under 15. This is not made perfectly clear in the text, and a specificity of close to zero is noted for a threshold of 15, which is clearly not true of the full dataset which, as seen above, is close to 80%.)

The area under the ROC curve for the above plot was calculated to be approximately 0.68. This means that 68% of the time a randomly selected patient from the pressure sore group has a higher Waterlow score than one from the no pressure sore group. It does not mean that a pressure sore occurs with a probability of 0.68, or that a pressure sore is associated with a positive result 68% of the time.[5]

Example: ROC analysis of radiograph assessment

Nurses and doctors were compared with respect to their ability to classify radiographs in an Accident and Emergency (A&E) department.[8] The X-ray assessor (junior doctor, experienced doctor, or nurse) stated how confident they are that a fracture was seen on an X-ray image. The gold standard used for the interpretation of the radiographs was the opinion of the consultant radiologist.

Using the gold standard to determine those images that did and did not show fractures, the sensitivity and specificity for each of five levels of confidence were calculated. An ROC analysis was used to compare the performance of nurses and doctors, and to compare junior doctors and experienced doctors. This analysis was used to determine whether it was appropriate for nurses to assess radiographs in the A&E department.

The radiological interpretations were recorded using an ascending rating scale of 1–5 which indicated the following confidence ratings (adapted from Zweig & Campbell[5]):

1 Definitely normal
2 Probably normal
3 Equivocal/suspicious/unclear
4 Probably abnormal
5 Definitely abnormal

Each subject was asked to indicate their responses to each of 50 radiographs using this scale. Through this process one was able to determine not just a positive or negative response to the findings, but also the degree of certainty with which that response was made. These aspects of the analysis are discussed in the following sections.

DRAWING THE ROC CURVE

For each threshold two parameters are measured: sensitivity and specificity (see Table 8.4). How to generate these values using SPSS will be discussed below.

The table may be used to draw the ROC plot (see Fig. 8.3). How such a graph can be created using SPSS is also discussed below. Note some workers use sensitivity against specificity, but most use (1 – specificity), which is the false positive rate. The two approaches are entirely analogous. Some ROC curves may be shown as percentages from 0% to 100% rather than as numbers 0 to 1; this is simply achieved by multiplying all the sensitivities and specificity figures by 100.

The better the classification the further the curve is from the diagonal. In a perfect classification all the patients below a certain threshold will have no fractures, and above it all the patients will have fractures. Ideally, data that are just above the threshold will give a point on the graph that is close to zero for the false positive rate and close to 100% for the true positive rate, i.e. a point that lies in the top left-hand corner of the graph and as far from the diagonal as possible.

In the real world there will usually be some incorrect classifications, but a good classification will have a threshold above which few false positives will be present but many true positives will be seen. Above the optimal threshold, the number of false positives will start to reduce, but less quickly than the number of true positives, and below the threshold the opposite will be true. Thus a curve is seen when plotting true against false positive (see Fig. 8.3). Two or more curves may be compared directly. If one curve lies above and to the left of the other it is a more accurate classifier (see Fig. 8.4, which shows that there is little difference between the performance of the nurses and the doctors).

USING SPSS TO PERFORM ROC ANALYSIS

SPSS does not have an ROC component. However, it is quite straightforward to perform an ROC analysis using SPSS built-in features. As an example, let us analyse the distal fracture radiograph data. In order to do the analysis we need the following information:

- The actual diagnosis (the gold standard), which we call 'goldstan', which is coded as 0 for no fracture and as 1 for a fracture
- The level of confidence with which the diagnosis is rated, we call this 'rating', which is coded from 5 (very confident disease is present) to 1 (very confident disease is not present)
- The profession of the assessor, which we will call 'profess', and code it as 1 for nurse and 2 for doctor.

In SPSS, we now use the Data pull-down menu and select Sort Cases. We then choose 'profess' in ascending order, then 'goldstan' in ascending order, and then 'rating' in descending order (Fig. 8.1). We obtain the data given in Table 8.1. Note that the number in the leftmost column is the row

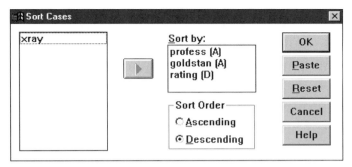

Figure 8.1 Sorting data: SPSS dialogue box.

Table 8.1   Data in SPSS spreadsheet ordered by 'profess' in ascending, 'goldstan' in ascending, and 'rating' in descending order

Number	goldstan	rating	profess
21	0	5	1
22	0	5	1
23	0	5	1
24	0	4	1
25	0	4	1

Table 8.2   As Table 8.1: last entries for false positives

Number	goldstan	rating	profess
180	0	1	1
181	0	1	1
182	0	1	1
183	0	1	1
184	0	1	1
185	1	5	1

(or record) number, i.e. the first record shown here is row 21 in the spreadsheet.

It can be seen that for profession code 1 (nurses), subject 23 scored their assessment of the (normal) radiograph as very confident for fracture, this is a false positive at a threshold of 5. If we move down the list (Table 8.2), we see that subject 184 scored with a confidence of 1 or above, which is all the diagnoses, as there is no threshold lower than 1. Note the record 185 is now a 'goldstan' of 1, i.e. a real fracture.

Intervening confidence levels can be read off by looking at where the

Table 8.3 As Table 8.1: false positives at a threshold of 4

Number	goldstan	rating	profess
62	0	4	1
63	0	4	1
64	0	4	1
65	0	4	1
66	0	3	1

Table 8.4 True positive rate and false positive rate for the diagnosis of distal fracture

Sensitivity (true positive rate)	1–Specificity (false positive rate)
0.75	0.13
0.88	0.35
0.89	0.46
0.97	0.78
1.00	1.00

'rating' changes. For example, in Table 8.3, subject 65 has a confidence level of 4.

As the total number of diagnoses is 184, the false positive rate at a threshold of 5 is $23/184 = 0.13$ (13%) and that at a threshold of 4 is $65/184 = 0.35$ (35%). The other values are easily computed (Table 8.4).

Re-ordering the data so that 'goldstan' is sorted in descending order we can similarly read off all the sensitivity readings. For example, the true positive rate at a threshold of 5 is seen to be $161/216$ (there are 216 diagnoses in total) or 0.75 (75%) (Table 8.5). This gives an immediate indication that the nurses are diagnosing rather than guessing, as the false positive rate was 13% at the same level. Again the calculation is repeated, at each threshold (see Table 8.4).

Placing the values for true and false positives for nurses into two new variables ntp and nfp, we can now get an ROC plot in SPSS by using the

Table 8.5 True positives at confidence level of 5

Number	goldstan	rating	profess
159	1	5	1
160	1	5	1
161	1	5	1
162	1	4	1
163	1	4	1

Graphs pull-down menu and selecting Scatter and then Simple. Place ntp on the y axis and nfp on the x axis. To give an optimal display, I forced the scales to lie within 0.0 and 1.0 for each axis by choosing Edit then Chart then Axis, and then selecting in turn each axis and setting the range of values to a minimum of 0.0 and a maximum of 1.0. See Figure 8.2, where the y axis is being set.

While still in the Edit mode, we can change the points to be a spline, which is easier to visualize, by clicking on the actual points, and selecting Attributes, then Interpolation, and then changing the default (None) to Spline. We get the graph shown in Figure 8.3.

Next we can perform the same analysis on the doctors, by re-sorting the data with 'profess' sorted in a descending manner. If the true and false positive rates for doctors are placed into new variables, say dtp and dfp, we can compare them directly with the nurses using the Overlay option in Scatter. We put the variables ntp and nfp as one pair, and dtp and dfp as the other pair. We can edit the graph as above, and then add grid lines to the plot by choosing Chart then Axis and, for each axis, x and y in turn, clicking on Grid in Major Division, setting the size of the division to our preferred value, say 0.1 for 10 lines (see Fig. 8.2 for the dialogue box that would be used). This will give a grid of 100 squares if both x and y axes are set to 10 divisions. Then we can count the squares under each line to give a measure of the area. A comparison of doctors and nurses is shown in Figure 8.4. The measurement of areas is often most easily achieved using a print-out. Alternatively, you could put the information

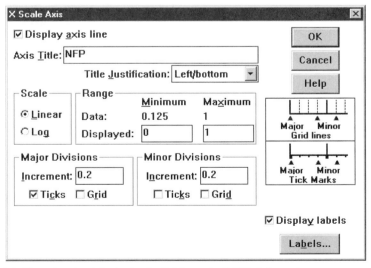

Figure 8.2 Changing the defaults for the ROC graph: SPSS dialogue box.

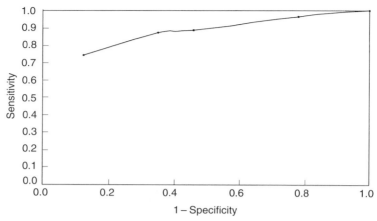

Figure 8.3 The ROC curve for the nurses' assessment of distal fractures.

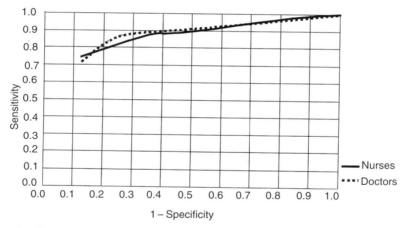

Figure 8.4 The ROC curves for the nurses' and doctors assessments of distal fractures.

into a spreadsheet program and calculate the area using the following algorithm:

$$\frac{\text{Area under curve between}}{\text{two successive points}} = \frac{\text{Mean value of two}}{\text{true positive scores}} \times \frac{\text{Difference of two}}{\text{false positive scores}}$$

Total area = Sum of successive individual areas

There are alternative methods for calculating the area under an ROC curve, and the above method will not give exactly the same value as that found by counting boxes under the spline, but should be the same as an

ROC plot obtained by interpolating with a straight line (which looks pretty horrid, hence my choice above). How you calculate the area is not critical, provided you used the same method throughout an analysis.

MEASURE OF CLASSIFICATION

The area under the curve gives some measure of the ability of the system to classify. An area of one-half of the maximum would be random (the area under the diagonal, which exactly splits the graph in two equal parts), while the nearer the value is to the maximum area the better the classification. One can use ROC to compare different classification systems directly. Examples might include:

- Two or more interpreters of a radiograph rating the presence of a fracture on a Likert scale (as in Figure 8.4)
- Two or more pressure sore risk scales
- Two or more clinicians diagnosing a disease
- Two or more automatic image analysis computer programs (as done by Anthony[13]).

COST

From an ROC plot we can obtain some idea of the best threshold to employ. If we look at pressure sore data (courtesy Pegasus Airwave), 69 patients from a population of 422 (or a ratio of 0.164) developed sores. The normal ratio is clearly 0.836. If we have already computed the sensitivity and specificity, then the overall error rate is

$$(1 - \text{Sensitivity})\,0.164 + (1 - \text{Specificity})\,0.836 = \text{Error}$$

which can be rearranged as

$$\text{Sensitivity} = \frac{(1 - \text{Specificity})\,0.836}{0.164} + c$$

where c is a constant. Then a series of lines of the form of the above equation, which differ only in the constant value c, can be drawn on the ROC curve.

Each of these lines has a gradient of 4.83, and the lowest value for the total error is found where one of these lines just touches the ROC curve. When the gradient is steep, a low sensitivity and high specificity is indicated; conversely, a shallow gradient indicates a high sensitivity and low specificity.

The above assumes that the cost of misclassifying (say) pressure sores as normal (false negative) is the same as misclassifying normals to be at risk of developing pressure sores (false positive). This is most unlikely. Suppose that the cost of misclassifying a normal patient as being at risk is the cost of a special mattress, and let us say for argument's sake that this involves a financial cost of £400 (this is a purely fictional number), but the cost of misclassifying a patient as normal when they go on to develop a sore is one month extra hospitalization, or (again purely fictional) a cost of £4000.

It can be shown that if the costs are L_1 for false positive and L_2 for false negative, the average cost is

Average cost = L_1 (1 – Specificity) 0.836 + L_2 (1 – Sensitivity) 0.164

So a similar set of equations to those above is created by the slight modification of including the cost values:

$$\text{Sensitivity} = \frac{(1 - \text{Specificity})0.836\,L_1}{0.164\,L_2} + c$$

Each line plotted according to the above equation has a gradient of $(0.836L_1)/(0.164L_2)$.

Thus increasing the cost L_1 will have the effect of increasing the gradient, and thus decreasing the sensitivity; and an increasing L_2 will increase sensitivity. In the present case the gradient will change from 4.83 to one-tenth of this value ($L_1/L_2 = 400/4000$) to 0.48. Figure 8.5 shows the ROC plot for these data, and two lines with gradients of approximately 4.8 and 0.48.

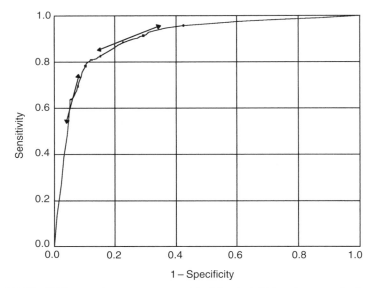

Figure 8.5 The ROC curve for pressure sore data. The straight lines have gradients of 4.8 and 0.48.

The former gives a sensitivity of about 0.65 and a specificity of about 0.95 (1 – Specificity = 0.05), i.e. a very low sensitivity and a high specificity. Therefore, many patients will be classified as normal who in fact go on to develop a sore. However, if the costs (here purely financial) are accounted for, the sensitivity goes up to about 0.9 and the specificity down to about 0.75 (1 – Specificity = 0.25). This would be achieved by lowering the threshold, in this case that in the Waterlow score.

Having said all the above, the main problem remains that of identifying the costs L_1 and L_2. The above gives financial costs, but what of the cost of pain and discomfort to the patient?

ADVANTAGES OF ROC

ROC has several advantages:

• ROC analysis allows you to assess a classification at several sensitivities and specificities, not merely one pair.
• Two or more ROC plots can be compared visually. A plot lying above and to the left of another plot shows greater accuracy.
• Sensitivity and specificity are calculated totally separately, using results from different groups. Sensitivity considers only those that have the condition, while specificity considers only those that do not. Thus the ROC plot is independent of prevalence of the disease (or condition under scrutiny, in the above cases fractures or sores).

PROBLEMS WITH ROC

ROC is not without its difficulties.

• Two ROC curves can have the same area but have very different characteristics. For example, one plot may have a much better specificity at low sensitivity, and the other better specificity at higher sensitivity.[5] The area under an ROC curve is a single measure, and information is necessarily lost by collapsing data down to one value. The whole plot should be examined.
• Relative costs of false classification (false positive and false negative) can be complex, so identifying the optimal threshold from an ROC plot is not necessarily easy. However, techniques do exist to achieve this end.[5]
• Comparison of ROC plots statistically can be difficult, especially where the tests are correlated (e.g. where two tests are performed on the same patient).

CONCLUSION

ROC is a useful method for assessing classification systems, and may be used to compare different classifiers quantitatively. It should be considered in audit and assessment tools that are numerical in nature and provide a clear output, but which are subject to probability rather than absolute certainty in the decision.

EXERCISES

1. Using the tables below, calculate the sensitivity and specificity of interpretations made by the casualty officers at a threshold above and equal to 'probably abnormal' (coded 4). Compare the values obtained with those for a threshold of 'abnormal'.

Sorted by 'profess' (descending), 'goldstan' (descending), and 'rating' (descending)

Number	goldstan	rating	profess
1	1	5	2
...	...	...	...
322	1	4	2
323	1	4	2
324	1	3	2
...	...	...	...
378	1	1	2
379	0	5	2

Sorted by 'profess' (descending), 'goldstan' (ascending), and 'rating' (descending)

Number	goldstan	rating	profess
1	0	5	2
...	...	...	...
76	0	4	2
77	0	4	2
78	0	3	2
...	...	...	...
322	0	1	2
323	1	5	2

2. Draw an ROC curve for the data given in the table above for Waterlow scores of over 15 given in Healy.[11] (Use SPSS if you have it; otherwise, use another statistics package, a spreadsheet or plot the curve by hand.) Calculate the area under the curve.

Waterlow score	Sensitivity	1 – Specificity
16	0.94	0.84
18	0.80	0.58
20	0.68	0.40
22	0.51	0.23
24	0.41	0.15
26	0.28	0.08

REFERENCES

1. Rose D 1995 Psychophysical methods. In: Breakwell G M, Hammond S, Fife-Schaw C (eds) Research methods in psychology. Sage, London
2. Swets J A 1979 ROC analysis applied to the evaluation of medical imaging techniques. Investigative Radiology 14(2): 109–121
3. Altman D G, Bland J M 1994 Diagnostic tests 1: sensitivity and specificity. British Medical Journal 308: 1552
4. Altman D G, Bland J M 1994 Diagnostic tests 3: receiver operating characteristic plots. British Medical Journal 309: 118
5. Zweig M H, Campbell G 1993 Receiver operating characteristic (ROC) plots: A fundamental evaluation tool in clinical medicine. Clinical Chemistry 39(40): 561–577
6. STEPS Consortium 1996 Medical screening, University of Glasgow, UK
7. Anthony D M 1996 A review of statistical methods in the *Journal of Advanced Nursing*. Journal of Advanced Nursing 24: 1089–1094
8. Overton P 1996 Towards a partnership in care: Nurses' and doctors' interpretation of extremity trauma radiology. Masters Thesis, University of Birmingham, UK
9. Cullum N, Dickson R, Eastwood A 1996 The prevention and treatment of pressure sores. Nursing Standard 26(10): 32–33
10. Waterlow J 1991 A policy that protects. Professional Nurse 6(5): 258–264
11. Healey F 1996 Waterlow revisited. Nursing Times 92(11): 80–84
12. Anthony D M 1996 Receiver operating characteristic analysis: An overview. Nurse Researcher 4(2): 75–88
13. Anthony D M 1991 The use of artificial neural networks in classifying lung scintigrams. PhD Dissertation, University of Warwick, UK

Principal components analysis and factor analysis

Measurements taken on a subject may be correlated. This means that there is a certain amount of redundancy in the data. In most real world problems there comes a point where adding a new variable tells us very little further about the subject. In extreme cases a variable may add no new information at all, in which case it is not necessary or even useful. However it is not always obvious which variables contain the most information. This chapter discusses methods of reducing data to the minimum number of variables, while keeping the maximum amount of information.

KEY POINTS

- Principal components analysis (PCA) is a special case of factor analysis (FA)
- PCA/FA is a method of reducing the number of variables or dimensions used to describe a dataset
- PCA/FA is typically used to explore data

At the end of this chapter the student should be able to:

1. Set up a dialogue box in SPSS to generate a PCA analysis

2. Interpret the output of an SPSS session for PCA/FA

INTRODUCTION

Principal components analysis (PCA) and the related method of factor analysis (FA) are methods of data reduction. A simple and straight-forward account is given by Hammond[1] and a more detailed introduction to its use in SPSS is given by Bryman & Cramer.[2] PCA is used to remove data that are either irrelevant or contain little useful information for the task at hand. It is best illustrated by an example.

Consider collecting data to describe the size of a human body. One could take a (potentially infinitely) large number of cross-sections, ending up with a huge data set that defines the individual body, but this is impractical in most situations. Thus one might choose anatomical lengths, or other data such as

1. left arm
2. right arm
3. left inside leg
4. right inside leg
5. head circumference
6. waist
7. chest
8. hips
9. weight
10. age
11. sex.

But do we need all these items? Data may be:

- *Redundant.* The left and right sides of the body are virtually the same, so why measure both?
- *Correlated.* Chest and waist size are correlated, so if you know one a plausible guess can be made for the other
- *Irrelevant.* Possibly age is not useful if we only consider adults.

If irrelevant redundant data are removed then no loss of accuracy occurs. If correlated data are removed some accuracy is lost, but this may be acceptable. PCA is a method by which data that are not working for us are removed.

PRINCIPAL COMPONENTS ANALYSIS

PCA and FA are used substantially in health care research. For example, in 6 months of the *Journal of Advanced Nursing* PCA/FA was used in several studies;[3] and examples from 1994 include the papers by Baggs,[4] Watson & Dreary,[5] Zhan & Shen,[6] van der Zee et al[7] and Fisher et al.[8]

There is some confusion in the texts between PCA and FA. The latter is a method of obtaining meaningful factors from a data set. These factors are produced by combining the variables of the original dataset, and are typically fewer in number than the original variables. PCA is one specific method of obtaining factors. It is the method favoured by most researchers using FA, but there are other methods. This chapter will concentrate on FA using principal components and, unless stated to the contrary, in this chapter the terms FA and PCA will be considered as synonymous (as is often the case in the literature).

PCA is related to correlation. In fact the analysis starts by producing a correlation matrix of all the variables. If two variables are highly correlated then one can probably be removed and still keep most of the information, as you can reconstitute the data by using regression. By this I mean that, as one variable seems to be largely predictable from another, you only need to keep one. For example, if a particular serum value A was almost always about twice another serum value B, then reporting both is largely unnecessary, because if you know B then $A = 2\,B$. You will only be able to get back all the lost data if the variables are totally correlated; however, a small loss of data is often acceptable, and an absolute correlation of less than 1.0 (i.e. > -1 and $< +1$) that is close to unity (i.e. much nearer to 1.0 than 0.0) may allow you to remove a variable with little loss of information. For example, a measurement of the left arm is likely to be very slightly different from one of the right arm, but we would accept either one, or the mean value of both as an accurate measure of arm length for most purposes.

As we saw in the chapter on partial correlation (Ch. 4) one variable may be partially correlated with several other variables. Thus a variable may not be strongly correlated with one variable, but is predictable from several taken together.

We usually view the variables in PCA as dimensions. This is analogous with spatial dimensions. Indeed the analogy is quite helpful in understanding PCA. I will now give some examples of physical dimensional systems (i.e. three-dimensional space, two-dimensional areas, one-dimensional lines), not because they are realistic representations of what we will perform PCA on, but because conceptually they are easy to understand. I will then extend the concept to other systems where the dimensions are not physical, but relate to any variables.

Suppose I am flying in a plane. To know my location you would need three dimensions: longitude, latitude and altitude. However, if I am sailing you would not need my altitude as it will always be (by the definition of sea level) zero. Thus my position is predicted from two dimensions: longitude and latitude. Now suppose I am driving along the M1 (a motorway linking London and the North of England, which passes near to my home Leicester) and I ask my passenger how far we are from home, they would only need one figure: the miles or kilometres to (in my case) Leicester. I still have three dimensions of travel, but only one is needed in this case, as the other two are constrained to be along the route of the motorway.

The above are pretty straightforward examples of dimension. However what if I were walking over the hilly park near my home. Assume you do not have a map with contours, if you knew my longitude and latitude very accurately you still do not know exactly where I am, as I may be up a hill or down a valley. However, your estimate of my exact position would be very close, as Leicestershire is not mountainous and, at most, I will be a couple of hundred metres away.

A further example is if you only had the time I had been gone to estimate where on a walk I might be. Since, from experience, you know I usually walk at a brisk rate of 3 miles per hour, you could use this to predict where I could be. However, you could be wrong for a variety of reasons, as I may walk a bit slower or faster, depending on the weather, my mood, etc. So time is correlated with distance, but the correlation is not entirely reliable. One could nevertheless use such a one-dimensional data set (time gone) to give an approximation of where I am. If I were known to stop for a pint in the village pub on the way home if I were thirsty, then knowing how thirsty I was to start with may add some useful information to the estimate of when I will return. However, it is possible that this information is not an accurate or sensitive measure, as it may be more dependent on who I see in the pub when I get there, which determines whether or not I stay.

The above examples are contrived and possibly rather silly, but are used to show:

• *A system may be underdefined*. If I want to describe a student's academic ability I may have several examination and course marks, but is it clear that I have enough? Suppose I only have one mark. It may not be representative of the student's work. This mark could be seen as one dimension of the student's work. This is a similar problem to only knowing when I left the house for my walk. However, even though the data are not ideal, they probably serve as the best estimate I have, and so are not useless.

• *A system may be overdefined*. Even if three dimensions are available, they are not necessarily all needed. This could be extended to any three (or any number of) variables, not just physical dimensions. In the student-assessment problem, I may have several marks from different courses and over many years. Therefore, adding another mark from a new assessed work may not make any difference to my assessment of the student, so why am I collecting such data?

• *The dimensions should be independent*. In working out a location in space, three properly chosen dimensions are needed. These are the three coordinates (length, breadth and height; or longitude, latitude and altitude). It is not possible to work out longitude from latitude or altitude, or any combination of these. If it were, then at least one dimension would be redundant, and could be disposed of.

In the sailing example, being given my altitude is useless as it is redundant as it will always be zero; a two-dimensional system (longitude and latitude) is equally as good as one that adds altitude. So if a parameter is constant, for example all the sample are of a similar age (e.g. a sample of first-year undergraduates), then the data on age are not likely to tell us anything extra. In the walking example, a two-dimensional system (longitude and latitude) is almost as good as the three-dimensional one. In the example where you only know how long I have been gone, a one-dimensional system (time) is a lot better than nothing, adding more data (thirst) helps, but may not be enough to be very useful. Thus, if we were paying for information, we would buy the time data, and only purchase the thirst data if it were very cheap.

A real-world example of data that is amenable to PCA analysis is compression of image data. There are many ways of reducing the amount of image data. You could simply send only half of the available data, which will give a more grainy image. However rather than simply throwing away half the data, you might try to work out which data contain the most information, and send the half (or some proportion) that contains the most. Images are divided into pixels, or points of light intensity. If an image is 100 pixels high and 100 pixels wide it contains 10 000 pixels, each of which can be viewed as a dimension. So we have 10 000 dimensions, where each dimension can be any value between (say) zero and 255. You could remove alternate rows and columns of pixels to reduce the data set, in this case to a quarter of the original size. You would probably get a better picture if you took some form of average of four adjacent points (in fact the median is usually used as it preserves lines better than the mean, this is known as *median filtering*). In this case we have reduced the dimensions from 10 000 to 2500, thus preserving (we hope) more information by combining the variables rather than simply throwing three-quarters of the data away. However, is median filtering optimal?

PCA would approach this problem by looking at the 10 000 dimensions of a sample of many pictures and work out what the correlations are among the pixels. It would then work out the best combination of variables to form a smaller number of new variables from the original data set that contain as much information as possible. This approach has been used in the analysis of medical images, for example in nuclear scintigrams.[9,10] In these studies the highly correlated scintigram images were used to produce a few variables, which in turn were used to create an automatic reporting system. PCA has also been used to reduce the number of inputs to a neural network (see Ch. 11). Neural networks scale badly, and therefore there is advantage in reducing the data set that is presented to the network, in order to keep the network as small as possible. Anthony and co-workers[11–13] have compared PCA with neural networks for data compression, and have used PCA to reduce the input data in a classification neural network. Neural networks with a reduced number of principal components performed better

> PCA is indicated when:
> - there are many variables that are correlated
> - the aim is to reduce the number of variables used to describe the data (i.e. when data compression is useful).

than those using raw data, even though some information was lost in the PCA reduction.

Technique

A correlation matrix is computed for all the variables that form the data set. It can be shown that a set of new variables, called *eigenvectors*, can be created that completely describe the correlation matrix, but these new variables are independent of each other (i.e. they are not correlated with each other). In a data set where some of the variables are totally redundant, the eigenvectors will be fewer in number than the original variables, but will contain exactly the same information. In general, however, for a data set with N variables, there will be, at most, N eigenvectors. The amount of information in each eigenvector, as measured by the amount of variance in the data set it describes, is not in general the same; some eigenvectors explain more variance than others, and may be said to contain more information.

Each eigenvector has an associated *eigenvalue*, which is the measure of the amount of variance in the data set it describes. If all the eigenvalues are summed, then the ratio of each eigenvalue to this sum is the percentage of the variance for which it accounts. Thus a sensible strategy for reducing the number of the variables in the data set is to take the first few eigenvectors with the highest eigenvalues. The algorithm for PCA can be described as follows:

1. Obtain eigenvectors of the correlation matrix
2. Arrange eigenvectors in decreasing order of their associated eigenvalues
3. Take the most important eigenvectors to describe the data.

While these steps can be achieved quite simply using mathematical packages such as Matlab, SPSS will do the analysis automatically for you. Select the Statistics menu in SPSS, then Data Reduction and then Factor.

Example: Examination marks

We have already looked at some examination marks in the chapter on ANOVA (Ch. 6). Suppose we want to know how many quantities we are actually assessing. We could count the number of subjects, or the number of course assignments and examinations. However, if several assignments measure the same thing, or if there is repetition between or among the subjects, this will not in general tell us how many items we are measuring.

Table 9.1 The 11 principal components of the marks for the nursing course

Variable name	Course
BIOL2	Biological science year 2
BRAN1_3	First branch-specific course year 3
BRAN1_4	First branch-specific course year 4
BRAN2_3	Second branch-specific course year 3
BRAN2_4	Second branch-specific course year 4
CHILD2	Child health year 2
MENTAL2	Mental health year 2
PHYSILL2	Physical illness year 2
PSYCH2	Psychology year 2
RESEAR3	Research methods and statistics year 3
RESEAR4	Research dissertation year 4

A factor analysis was computed using principal components of the marks for the nursing course, which are listed in Table 9.1. We can think of these as the 11 dimensions of the data, which we wish to reduce if possible.

SPSS, by default, shows only eigenvalues over 1.0 (*Kaiser's criterion*). The logic for this is that the sum of the eigenvalues is equal to the original number of variables, and therefore any eigenvector with an eigenvalue under unity is accounting for, on average, less than the original variable (otherwise, the SPSS default settings were used in this analysis). However, this retention criterion has been criticized as having no scientific basis.[2] Using SPSS with all 11 eigenvectors being reported gave the output shown in Figure 9.1.

In the default setting, the FA is computed using principal components (there are

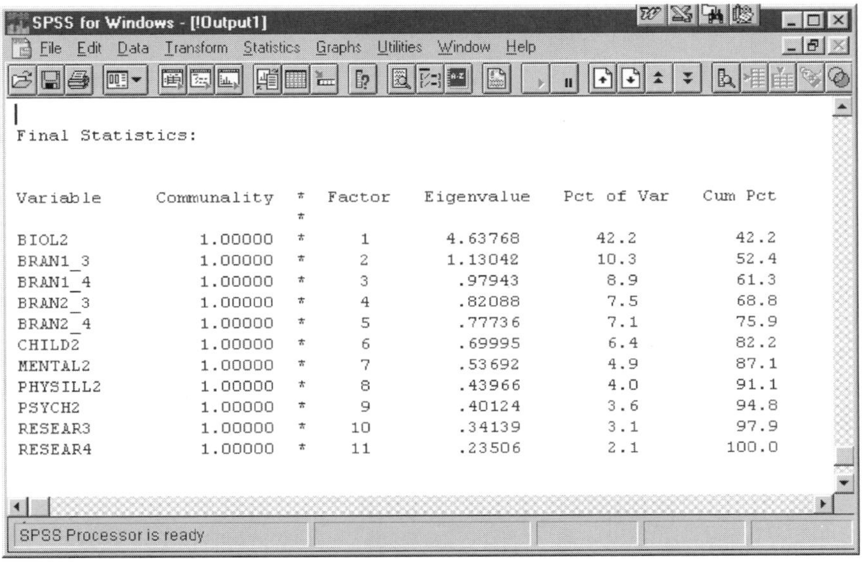

```
Final Statistics:

Variable     Communality  *  Factor  Eigenvalue  Pct of Var  Cum Pct
                          *
BIOL2          1.00000    *    1       4.63768      42.2       42.2
BRAN1_3        1.00000    *    2       1.13042      10.3       52.4
BRAN1_4        1.00000    *    3        .97943       8.9       61.3
BRAN2_3        1.00000    *    4        .82088       7.5       68.8
BRAN2_4        1.00000    *    5        .77736       7.1       75.9
CHILD2         1.00000    *    6        .69995       6.4       82.2
MENTAL2        1.00000    *    7        .53692       4.9       87.1
PHYSILL2       1.00000    *    8        .43966       4.0       91.1
PSYCH2         1.00000    *    9        .40124       3.6       94.8
RESEAR3        1.00000    *   10        .34139       3.1       97.9
RESEAR4        1.00000    *   11        .23506       2.1      100.0
```

Figure 9.1   PCA/FA of nursing course marks: SPSS Output screen.

other methods, which we will not discuss here). The SPSS output shows the variables used in the first column, then the *communality* (discussed below). The next columns are used to show the 11 eigenvalues of the eigenvectors. These eigenvectors are not (in general) original variables, but are created as combinations of the original variables. I stress this as it is easy to make the mistake of looking across the row and assuming that the first row (for example) gives the first eigenvalue (which it does) and that this is the eigenvalue of BIOL2 (which it is not). The original variables are simply shown in alphabetical order, and are totally separate from the right-hand part of the display, which shows the eigenvalues. Thus the display in Figure 9.1 shows that the particular combination of the original variables makes up the most important eigenvector, with an eigenvalue of about 4.64, accounting for 42.2% of the variance.

SPSS then goes on to show you the eigenvectors (factors), summarized in Table 9.1, and the correlations of each variable with each factor. For example, the first two in this example are given in Table 9.2. If we consider that the data are adequately described by factors 1 and 2, then we have succeeded in reducing the data to two dimensions.

It is common to use one of two methods to interpret the values given:[2]

1. Ignore those absolute correlation values that are small, conventionally under 0.3 (as these account for only 9% of the variance).

2. Ignore values that 'load on' more than one factor, as this results in each factor consisting of variables that are unique to it. For example, RESEAR4 has values above 0.3 on both factor 1 and factor 2, and we would therefore say it is not unique to either of these factors.

Using rule 1, factor 1 is simply representative of all variables (all correlations being reasonably high), and could be said to be simply measuring overall ability in taking examinations. Factor 2 seems to be associated mainly with research skills. In this case rule 2 is not very helpful, except that is could be interpreted as removing research skills from factor 1.

Table 9.2 The correlations between the first two eigen vectors (factors) and the 11 variables

	Factor 1	Factor 2
BIOL2	**0.65148**	0.07538
BRAN1_3	**0.58569**	−0.00069
BRAN1_4	**0.71836**	**−0.30979**
BRAN2_3	**0.75000**	0.07110
BRAN2_4	**0.56824**	−0.02409
CHILD2	**0.56999**	−0.056496
MENTAL2	**0.61948**	0.13962
PHYSILL2	**0.78707**	−0.33112
PSYCH2	**0.66819**	0.17644
RESEAR3	**0.71209**	**0.31451**
RESEAR4	**0.43257**	**0.66691**

Bold numbers indicate meaningful variables.

To aid interpretation, SPSS allows factors to be *rotated* in a variety of ways. To explain the concept of rotation, think of the simple two-factor/two-dimension situation which can be visualized as a graph with two axes at right angles (*orthogonal*) to each other. These axes (each representing a factor) can be constructed in different ways, moved into different positions, or rotated, to make the resulting factors more easily interpretable. The *Varimax* rotation is the method used to simplify the interpretation of factors. Using Kaiser's criterion and the Varimax rotation we get two variables, as shown in Figure 9.2 and Table 9.3.

The interpretation of the above is similar, in that by rule 1 (correlations < 0.3) research is now excluded from factor 1, and factor 2 is now loading on most

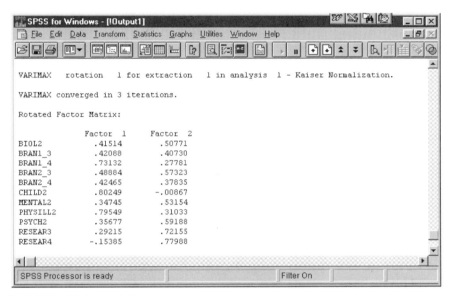

Figure 9.2   Varimax rotation.

Table 9.3 Factors 1 and 2 rotated using Kaiser's criterion and the Varimax rotation

	Factor 1	Factor 2
BIOL2	**0.41514**	**0.50771**
BRAN1_3	**0.42088**	**0.40730**
BRAN1_4	**0.73132**	0.27781
BRAN2_3	**0.48884**	**0.57323**
BRAN2_4	**0.42465**	**0.37835**
CHILD2	**0.80249**	−0.00867
MENTAL2	**0.34745**	**0.53154**
PHYSILL2	**0.79549**	**0.31033**
PSYCH2	**0.35677**	**0.59188**
RESEAR3	0.29215	**0.72155**
RESEAR4	−0.15385	**0.77988**

Bold numbers indicate meaningful variables.

variables. Factor 1 could be said to be non-research skills, and factor 2 an overall ability in examinations, but especially research. Rule 2 would indicate that factor 2 is a research factor, and factor 1 is concerned with branch-specific courses (BRAN1_4 and CHILD2).

Yet another way to rotate the variables is via an *oblique rotation*, this is alleged to allow easier interpretation of the variables, but produces factors that are not necessarily independent of each other. This method is used as it is argued that the orthogonal rotation used by Varimax may produce factors that are not very realistic. Table 9.4 shows an oblique rotation on this data. (SPSS gives a pattern and structure matrix. We usually use the structure matrix, which consists of the correlations of each of the variables with the factors; but in the orthogonal rotation the two matrices are identical and only the structure matrix is shown. See Figure 9.3.)

Using rule 1 again, factor 1 shows overall ability, and factor 2 features the research dissertation and two of the second year courses. Rule 2 would appear to allow no interpretation of factor 2.

There is considerable debate about the relative merits of the different rotations, but it would seem to be the case that whatever method we use we are seeing that the largest component of the variance of the data is overall ability, and the next most important are the skills shown especially in the dissertation. This is unsurprising, as the dissertation is not assessed by examination, whereas all the other courses are. However, there is some indication that the research (examinable) course in year 3 should be grouped with the dissertation, so we may be seeing ability to use (say) statistics as the relevant item that groups these components together. It should be stressed that FA is being used here in an exploration of the data, and thus the ideas it is throwing up may be used for further analysis. We have not proved that research really is different from the other parts of the curriculum, although it is not an unreasonable suggestion.

The communality of the variables is defined as the variance of the variables accounted for by the factors identified. Using Kaiser's criterion with an oblique

Table 9.4 Factors 1 and 2 rotated using an oblique rotation

	Factor 1	Factor 2
BIOL2	**0.65565**	−0.03681
BRAN1_3	**0.58315**	−0.10055
BRAN1_4	**0.68687**	−0.42775
BRAN2_3	**0.75336**	−0.05784
BRAN2_4	**0.56363**	−0.12064
CHILD2	**0.51569**	**−0.65388**
MENTAL2	**0.62969**	0.03193
PHYSILL2	**0.75333**	**−0.46048**
PSYCH2	**0.68157**	0.05992
RESEAR3	**0.73796**	0.18848
RESEAR4	**0.49200**	**0.58338**

Bold numbers indicate meaningful variables.

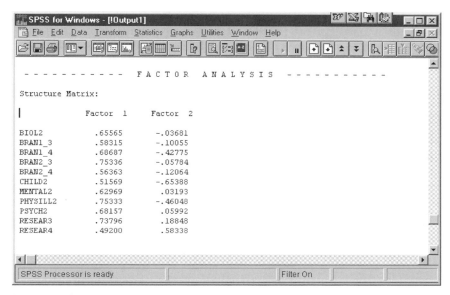

Figure 9.3   Structure matrix for oblique rotation.

Table 9.5 Communality between factors 1 and 2 and the 11 variables

Variable	Communality*	Factor	Eigenvalue	Pct of Var	Cum Pct
BIOL2	0.43011*	1	4.63768	42.2	42.2
BRAN1_3	0.34303*	2	1.13042	10.3	52.4
BRAN1_4	0.61201*				
BRAN2_3	0.56756*				
BRAN2_4	0.32348*				
CHILD2	0.64406*				
MENTAL2	0.40325*				
PHYSILL2	0.72912*				
PSYCH2	0.47761*				
RESEAR3	0.60598*				
RESEAR4	0.63189*				

rotation, for example, gives two factors. Table 9.5 identifies for our two factors how much variance (as a proportion) of each variable is accounted for. It is seen that all variables have 32–72% of the variance accounted for by just two of the 11 possible factors. Adding another three factors explains more variance (in fact the figures go up to 66–88%).

Example: Waterlow scores in hospital patients

I am grateful to Dr Michael Clarke of Pegasus who gave me access to the hospital data used in this example.

The Waterlow score, which is used to assess the risk of pressure sore occurrence, is composed of 11 subscores, but has never been formally evaluated by regression analysis, nor has the relevance of the subscores been rigorously assessed.[14] One way to look at these data is to see how much variance is accounted for by each variable, and to see whether combining the variables would retain most of the data. This might indicate which variables are worth serious consideration.

Performing a straightforward PCA factor analysis on the 11 components (it is coincidental that both this and the previous example contain 11 variables) listed in Table 9.6 gives the factors listed in Table 9.7.

Note that the first factor accounts for 21% and the last factor for 4%, so the first factor seems to be about five times as important as the last. As discussed above there is some controversy about how best to identify the number of factors to be used. One method, available in SPSS, is a scree chart. This plots the eigenvalues in descending order. The idea is that if the data set is inherently (for example) three-dimensional, and we are simply collecting the other eight variables unnecessarily, then all the information will be in the first three eigenvectors

Table 9.6 The 11 principal components of the Waterlow score

Variable	Description
WATAGE	Age
WATAPPET	Appetite
WATBUILD	Body Build
WATCON	Continence
WATMED	Medication
WATMOBIL	Mobility
WATNEURO	Neurological deficit
WATSEX	Gender
WATSKIN	State of the skin
WATSURG	Recent surgery
WATTMAL	Tissue malnutrition

Table 9.7 The factors obtained from the analysis of the 11 components of the Waterlow score

Factor	Eigenvalue	Pct of Var	Cum Pct
1	**2.34071**	**21.3**	**21.3**
2	**1.38829**	**12.6**	**33.9**
3	**1.12387**	**10.2**	**44.1**
4	**1.09392**	**9.9**	**54.1**
5	**1.01045**	**9.2**	**63.2**
6	0.86514	7.9	71.1
7	0.77943	7.1	78.2
8	0.71935	6.5	84.7
9	0.66712	6.1	90.8
10	0.55647	5.1	95.9
11	0.45525	4.1	100.0

Bold numbers indicate meaningful variables.

(factors). In the real world, of course, there will be random errors (often called noise, especially in engineering circles) and the three first factors will not account for all the variance in the given data set. However, random errors are argued to produce eigenvectors that have similar eigenvalues to each other, and the scree plot should thus level out. Therefore you should look for where the plot becomes flat and ignore all factors beyond that point.

In SPSS, selecting Extraction from the Factor dialogue box allows you to elect to produce a scree plot (Fig. 9.4) and also to change the default behaviour of using Kaiser's criterion. In the present case I have chosen to use all 11 factors. Figure 9.5 shows the scree plot, and it could be argued that it shows the first three factors as useful. The next two factors have an eigenvalue of over unity, and would under Kaiser's criterion be kept; however, they are borderline as both are under 1.1. Between them however the variance accounted for increases from 44% (three factors) to 63% (five factors), and thus they might be worth keeping.

If we look at the correlations of the variables with the factors (Table 9.8), we can, using the rules outlined above, see that interpretation is not easy. Using rule

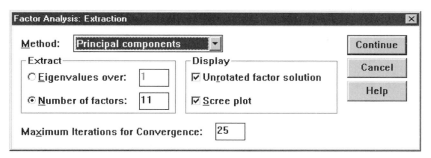

Figure 9.4   Factor analysis: SPSS Extraction dialogue box.

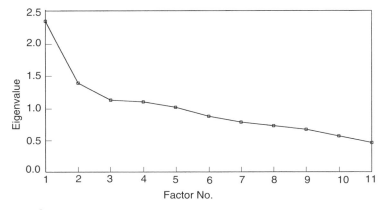

Figure 9.5   Scree plot.

Table 9.8 Correlations between the 11 variables and factors 1–5

	Factor 1	Factor 2	Factor 3	Factor 4	Factor 5
WATAGE	**0.67860**	−0.30367	−0.15133	0.05064	−0.15328
WATAPPET	**0.43268**	**0.35041**	0.28809	0.09467	0.18712
WATBUILD	**0.42691**	−0.28220	0.12118	**0.50452**	0.15172
WATCON	**0.45629**	**0.48634**	−0.16943	−0.15536	0.19205
WATMED	−0.17436	−0.17941	0.03044	0.13237	**0.90872**
WATMOBIL	**0.71420**	0.10677	0.04699	−0.25991	−0.00452
WATNEURO	0.19374	**0.48767**	**0.57494**	−0.24079	0.05871
WATSEX	**0.32042**	0.27545	−0.15883	**0.65760**	−0.14369
WATSKIN	**0.73323**	−0.30385	−0.01454	−0.05124	0.03868
WATSURG	0.19769	0.09883	−0.71755	**−0.34426**	0.20153
WATTMAL	0.21249	**−0.63067**	**0.31712**	**−0.32723**	−0.00570

Bold numbers indicate meaningful variables.

1, and working backwards from factor 5, seems to be explicable by medication alone (hence an eigenvalue of near 1). Factor 4 is difficult to make much sense of, unless there is some logical relationship between build, gender, surgery and tissue malnutrition. I could construct such a relationship; we know that patients who have had surgery are often malnourished, especially if they have had gastrointestinal surgery, and this should have an effect on build. However, why is gender relevant here? Tissue malnutrition includes smoking as an item, possibly gender is a proxy for smoking or other items in the tissue malnutrition variable. I could further postulate that smoking will cause you to undergo more surgery for smoking-related disease. Maybe factor 4 is a smoking factor. However, we have proved nothing with this chain of thought, and further analysis will be needed. Factor 3 is predominantly neurological deficit (paraplegia, cerebrovascular accident (CVA), etc.) and tissue malnutrition (as recorded by the presence of anaemia, smoking, cardiac failure, etc.), so this might also be a smoking factor, with smoking leading to higher chances of circulatory disease such as CVA, which is known to be true. Factor 3 could, alternatively, be said to be an indicator of disorders that put a patient at special risk. Factors 1 and 2 are again difficult to make sense of.

Using rule 2, we can rearrange the meaningful variables as shown in Table 9.9. It again seems that medication is the relevant item for factor 5, surgery for factor 4, and mobility for factor 1; factors 2 and 3 are not interpretable using rule 2. Thus we see that FA/PCA does not necessarily give us intuitively easy interpretations of the factors.

Example: Waterlow on wheelchair patients

I am grateful to Dr Jim Unsworth, consultant of the West Midlands Rehabilitation Clinic, for access to this dataset, which comprised part of a Masters thesis by one of my students.[15]

Table 9.9 Rearrangement of the meaningful variables shown in Table 9.8

	Factor 1	Factor 2	Factor 3	Factor 4	Factor 5
WATAGE	0.67860	−0.30367	−0.15133	0.05064	−0.15328
WATAPPET	0.43268	0.35041	0.28809	0.09467	0.18712
WATBUILD	0.42691	−0.28220	0.12118	0.50452	0.15172
WATCON	0.45629	0.48634	−0.16943	−0.15536	0.19205
WATMED	−0.17436	−0.17941	0.03044	0.13237	**0.90872**
WATMOBIL	**0.71420**	0.10677	0.04699	−0.25991	−0.00452
WATNEURO	0.19374	0.48767	0.57494	−0.24079	0.05871
WATSEX	0.32042	0.27545	−0.15883	0.65760	−0.14369
WATSKIN	0.73323	−0.30385	−0.01454	−0.05124	0.03868
WATSURG	0.19769	0.09883	−0.71755	**−0.34426**	0.20153
WATTMAL	0.21249	−0.63067	0.31712	−0.32723	−0.00570

Bold numbers indicate meaningful variables

The factors found in the Waterlow scores for hospital patients may show different loadings if applied to another domain. Clearly hospital patients are quite likely, for example, to have had an operation, so the variables that deal with surgery will show variance. However, a cohort of wheelchair users will not typically have had recent surgery. Thus, even though surgery may be a useful predictor of complications (such as pressure sores) in general, it will not necessarily contain much useful information about this new group.

If we use the same variables as in the above example, then the output of the FA/PCA (using PCA and all factors being retained) is as shown in Figure 9.6. The

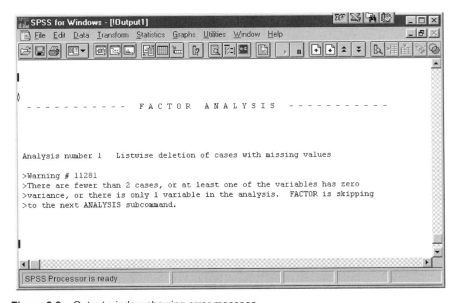

Figure 9.6 Output window showing error message.

Table 9.10 Correlations between the 10 variables and factors 1–5: wheelchair users

	Factor 1	Factor 2	Factor 3	Factor 4	Factor 5
WATAGE	**0.59849**	−0.10072	**0.50514**	−0.18468	0.22408
WATAPPET	**0.51149**	0.25426	0.16020	**0.46381**	0.03724
WATBUILD	**0.31483**	**0.60908**	**0.30286**	−0.13033	0.29557
WATMED	0.14763	**−0.52834**	**0.49587**	**−0.42942**	−0.22121
WATMOBIL	**−0.67407**	**0.33576**	0.08652	0.18557	−0.06101
WATNEURO	**−0.75045**	0.13803	−0.15051	**0.32255**	−0.05818
WATSEX	**0.48260**	**0.31107**	**−0.40018**	−0.00615	−0.29445
WATSKIN	−0.07317	−0.06942	**0.72790**	**0.43416**	0.05502
WATTMAL	0.09517	**−0.32013**	−0.20467	0.05252	**0.86790**
WATCON	0.13181	**0.72428**	0.15939	−0.29022	0.07458

Bold numbers indicate meaningful variables.

error message was caused by (at least) one of the variables having no variance at all; thus no factors could be computed. Removing the relevant variable, recent surgery (WATSURG), gives the factors shown in Table 9.10.

By either rule, the factors seem to be composed of different variables than those generated by the hospital cases. Using rule 2, for example, only continence is relevant, a variable not seen in the previous FA/PCA analysis, and accounting for factor 2. Using rule 1, factor 5 is now special risk items for tissue malnutrition (WATTMAL), whereas before it was medication.

CONCLUSION

PCA/FA is a method of reducing the number of variables in a dataset while keeping as much information as possible. It may be used to:

- reduce the amount of data that is needed
- to explore possible factors in a dataset.

It is not necessarily the case that the factors identified are, in general, those most useful; rather the factors identified are simply those that describe the data to hand. It is possible that an analysis using PCA/FA on new data will give different results (i.e. the analysis results are not necessarily generalizable), and therefore caution should be employed in interpreting the results, especially if the new data are not from a similar population. Thus the factors for Waterlow scores from wheelchair patients are not likely to be the same as those for scores from hospital patients, and may not be similar even to those for another cohort of wheelchair users.

As an exploratory technique PCA/FA has merits in identifying plausible factors in the data that may be analysed by other methods. It can be used in qualitative analysis, and thus we may remove some of the more rigid restrictions, such as insisting on using normal data, provided we treat the results with appropriate caution.

If factors are shown to be generalizable then they may be used to compress data. For example, the principal components of a dataset may be employed to compress another similar dataset (i.e. not one on which the PCA was computed) and an estimate of the original data can be computed by restoring the reduced dataset back to the original number of variables using an inverse matrix of the PCA matrix. This can be compared with the original data to see how well it has restored the data. If it is similar to the accuracy of the restoration of the data used to compute the principal components, then the PCA is considered to have generalized. This is similar to the notion of neutral networks (see Ch. 11) having learned the 'right' solution.

EXERCISE

1. An analysis was made of the death rates of young adult males aged 20–24 years (DEA20_24), three measures of mortality in the very young (infant mortality, INFORMT; neonatal mortality, NEONATAL; and perinatal mortality, PERINAT) and gross domestic product per capita (GDP) for many countries in Europe. The default behaviour of extracting principal components with eigenvalues over 1.0 was employed, with no rotation. Using the output data shown below, answer the following questions:

   (a) How many factors would be needed to account for at least 90% of the variance of the data.

   (b) Using the two techniques discussed in the text, identify the variables that are relevant to factors 1 and 2.

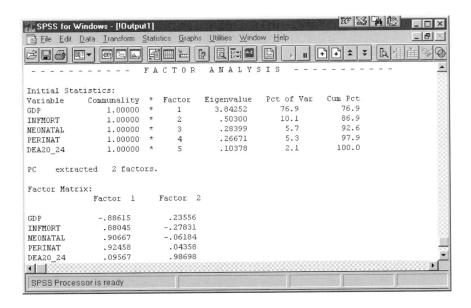

(c) Interpret the meaning of the factors.
(d) Changing the default behaviour of SPSS to obtain all factors, factor 3 was found to be:

GDP	0.39320
INFMORT	−0.07512
NEONATAL	0.18278
PERINAT	0.27276
DEA20_24	−0.10886

Interpret this third factor.

REFERENCES

1. Hammond S 1995 Introduction to multivariate data analysis. In: Brakwell G M, Hammond S, Fife-Schaw C (eds) Research methods in psychology. Sage, London, p 360–385
2. Bryman A, Cramer D 1997 Quantitative data analysis. Routledge, London, p 276–291
3. Anthony D M 1996 A review of statistical methods in the *Journal of Advanced Nursing*. Journal of Advanced Nursing 24: 1089–1094
4. Baggs J 1994 Development of an instrument to measure collaboration and satisfaction about care decisions. Journal of Advanced Nursing 20 (1): 176–182
5. Watson R, Deary I 1994 Measuring feeding difficulty in patients with dementia-multivariate-analysis of feeding problems nursing intervention and indicators of feeding difficulty. Journal of Advanced Nursing 20 (2): 283–287
6. Zhan L, Shen C 1994 The development of an instrument to measure self-consistency. Journal of Advanced Nursing 20 (2): 509–516
7. van der Zee, Kramer K, Derksen A, Kerkstra A, Stevens F C J 1994 Community nursing in Belgium, Germany and the Netherlands. Journal of Advanced Nursing 20 (5): 791–801
8. Fisher M L, Hinson N, Deets C 1994 Selected predictors of registered nurses' intent to stay. Journal of Advanced Nursing 20 (5): 950–957
9. Barber D C 1980 The use of principal components in the quantitative analysis of gamma camera dynamic studies. Physics in Medicine and Biology 25 (2): 283–292
10. Barber D C, Nijran K S 1985 Towards automatic analysis of dynamic radionuclide studies using principal components analysis. Physics in Medicine and Biology 30 (12): 1315–1325
11. Anthony D M 1991 The use of artificial neural networks in classifying lung scintigrams. PhD dissertation, University of Warwick, UK
12. Anthony D M, Barham J, Hines E L, Taylor D 1990 A comparison of image compression by neural networks and principal components analysis. In: Proceedings of the 4th international joint conference on neural networks. IEEE, San Diego, 3: 339–344
13. Anthony D M, Barham J, Hines E L, Taylor D 1989 A study of data compression using neural networks and principal component analysis. In: IEE coloquium on biomedical applications of digital signal processing. IEE, London, p 2/1–2/4.
14. Cullum N, Dickson R, Eastwood A 1996 The prevention and treatment of pressure sores. Nursing Standard 26 (10): 32–33
15. Barnes J 1997 Prevention of pressure sores in community-based wheelchair users. A study examining the use of risk calculators and the relevance of risk factors to assess pressure sore risk in community-based wheelchair users. Masters thesis, University of Birmingham, UK

Cluster analysis and discriminant analysis

We try to comprehend the world by classifying items into categories. For example the animal kingdom is split into mammals, reptiles, insects etc. These categories are themselves capable of further refinement, so mammals are split into dogs, cats, horses etc. This chapter describes some methods for classifying data.

KEY POINTS

- Cluster analysis is a method of exploring data
- A metric is a measure of how far apart two items are
- Clustering can simply split items into clusters at the same level, or place them in a hierarchical structure
- Discriminant analysis apportions items into groups

At the end of this chapter the student should be able to:

1. Use SPSS to undertake a cluster analysis or discriminant analysis

2. Interpret dendrograms and icicle plots

3. Interpret the discriminant equation

INTRODUCTION

This purpose of this chapter is to discuss two methods of categorizing data, cluster and discriminant analysis, both of which appear in the Professional Statistics part of the SPSS package.

A method of splitting the data into natural clusters is named cluster analysis. The aim of cluster analysis is to investigate the underlying structure of the data. The first section of this chapter will describe cluster analysis. For a fuller treatment on cluster analysis see Everitt.[1]

Suppose we are presented with a set of data, and wish to describe its characteristics. For example, the Waterlow score (see Chs 8 and 9) identifies 11 variables, which are designed to differentiate those patients who will develop pressure sores from those who will not. Thus implicit in the Waterlow score is a structure of two groups: sore and no sore. We could refer to a 'cluster' of patients with sores and a cluster with no sores. However, does the Waterlow score naturally split into two clusters such as these? Using one form of cluster analysis, where the number of clusters is given (here 2), we can explore whether the scoring system inherently falls into the required clusters. Later in this chapter there is an example which looks at such a clustering problem.

However, not all problems are as simple as classification into two, or very few, groups. Cluster analysis deals with more complex relationships, which could include subgroups of groups, and it is concerned with showing the structure of the data. For example, life on Earth could be split into the animal kingdom, the plant kingdom and fungi, and micro-organisms (bacteria, viruses). Animals can be further split into chordates (having a backbone) and several other phyla, for example echinoderms (starfish, etc.). These large categories can be split into smaller ones, for example mammals are part of the chordates and reptiles are another group.

There are two ways of performing a hierarchical cluster analysis. One method is to group variables, the idea here being to decide which variables are close to each other and how the variables group together. In the second method, individuals in the sample are placed into clusters. Later in this chapter an example is given of each of these ways of doing a cluster analysis.

Individuals can be allocated into groups (or clusters) on the basis of how 'close' they are to each other. We would naturally say that pigs are closer to humans than, say, crocodiles. But apes are closer to humans than pigs. But on what basis is this measure of 'closeness' made? One measure would be the percentage of DNA each species has in common. If, for example, on this basis chimpanzees and humans were 95% the same, and some other ape was 90% the same as humans, then we would say that chimpanzees were closer to humans than some other ape (say orang-utans). It is noted that a different from of measuring closeness might give a totally different taxonomy. Suppose we have features that measure how an animal feeds, humans might then be seen as very close to pigs (both omnivores) and more different from gorillas (strict vegetarians). Thus the taxonomy is highly dependent on our measures (called *metrics*) which should be chosen to identify the feature of interest, which itself may not be straightforward or obvious.

We could put humans, chimps and other apes in one cluster (primates), and dogs, pigs, cats and horses in other clusters. These all fit into a super-cluster (mammals) and all mammals along with reptiles and most fish go into chordates, which themselves go with elasmobranches (sharks) and echinoderms into the animal kingdom, which is quite separate from, say, bacteria. Finally, even bacteria and humans are related, as they have a common ancestor (something like algae about 3.5 billion years ago). If life were to be found on Mars, it would probably be even further removed from us than bacteria. This form of clustering is hierarchical, in the sense that not only are there different groups (clusters) but there is also a natural ordering and depth of clusters and relationships between clusters.

A different but related concept to clustering is that of *discrimination*. So we might want to discriminate between those patients who will develop a sore, and those who will not. In Chapters 7 and 11 we have seen some methods of attempting to predict one variable from one or more other variables, and discriminant analysis is another such technique. It is based on the assumption that there is a linear relationship between the variables. For a fuller treatment of discriminant analysis see Lachenbroch.[2]

Texts that contain some material on cluster and discriminant analysis include those by Cooley & Lohnes,[3] Gorsuch[4] and Manly.[5] A straightforward account of these techniques can be found in Hammond.[6] For a good text on both these types of analysis specifically for SPSS see Norusis.[7]

Discriminant analysis and cluster analysis both place cases into classes. They can be used in similar applications as principal component analysis (PCA) and factor analysis (FA) to identify the groupings within a data set. Both discriminant and cluster analysis can be used in exploratory data analysis. Where they differ is that cluster analysis is more concerned with showing the structure of a dataset, while discriminant analysis places cases into previously identified categories.

CLUSTER ANALYSIS

Cluster analysis is used to group individual cases into discrete groups. It uses some method of determining how close two individuals are (the *metric* or distance, see below) and individuals that are close to each other based on this metric are said to be in same group. Grouping can be:

- *In a cascade, or hierarchy, or taxonomy.* All items belong in one super-ordinate or general group, which is broken down into smaller and smaller subgroups. The investigator does not state how many groups there are. Example, the animal kingdom.
- *Non-hierarchical.* The investigator states how many groups there are and the program assigns items to groups depending on how similar they are to each other. For example, the 11 variables in the Waterlow score.

The investigator may need to state the number of clusters that will be found, and this should be done on a theoretical basis. The investigator will also need to be able to interpret the clusters once they have been located, and this can be difficult.

Cluster analysis is typically used for exploration of data, and tasks suitable to cluster analysis include:

- finding a typology
- model fitting
- prediction based on groups
- hypothesis testing
- hypothesis generation
- data reduction.

Hierarchical methods

Data are not partitioned into groups in one go, but are grouped into broad classes, which are then classified into smaller groups. The method typically used is agglomerative, whereby cases that are near to each other are placed in the same cluster. The distances between the clusters may then be calculated, and nearer clusters are placed in superclusters, etc. The algorithm is as follows:

1. Compute differences between items
2. Fuse items that are nearest
3. Go to step 1 until all items or subgroups are in one large group.

There are several options about how to merge items or clusters. In *nearest neighbour clustering*, groups are fused according to the distance between nearest neighbours, i.e. close cases or clusters are put together. In *centroid clustering*, groups are depicted as lying in Euclidean space, and a group is said to lie where the centroid of the group lies. *Median clustering* is where groups are merged, and the new position is the median of the values of the old groups.

Metrics

If clusters are formed by merging close members, there has to be a measure of what closeness is. A metric is a measure of how close (or far apart) two individuals are. Metrics have the following features, where $d(x,y)$ is the distance between x and y:

- $d(x,y) \geq 0$: the distance between x and y is either zero or positive (like ordinary distances); in particular, $d(x,y) = 0$ implies $x = y$, and vice versa. If the distance between two objects is zero, they must be in the same place.
- $d(x,y) = d(y,x)$: the distance between x and y is the same as the distance between y and x.

- $d(x,y) + d(y,z) \geqslant d(x,z)$: the distance between x and y added to the distance between y to z can never be more than the distance between x and z.

There are many metrics, but typically the *simple Euclidean distance coefficient* is used. For one dimension (variable), with two values x_1 and x_2, this is just the distance

$$d = x_1 - x_2$$

For two dimensions, with values (x_{11}, x_{12}) and (x_{21}, x_{22}), this is the pythagorus distance

$$d = \sqrt{[(x_{11}-x_{21})^2 + (x_{12}-x_{22})^2]}$$

For three dimensions, with values (x_{11}, x_{12}, x_{13}) and (x_{21}, x_{22}, x_{23}):

$$d = \sqrt{[(x_{11}-x_{21})^2 + (x_{12}-x_{22})^2 + (x_{13}-x_{23})^2]}$$

In general, with n dimensions, two items could be measured in n dimensions. That is, n variables are used to represent each item. In three-dimensional space this would be x,y,z coordinates, but equally a patient may have three blood measurements which could be combined to reach a diagnosis. Two points in space or two patients each with three blood test measurements would both be represented as x_{11}, x_{12}, x_{13} and x_{21}, x_{22}, x_{23}. Extending the concept to an arbitrary number of dimensions, and calling this number n, where n could be 3 for the examples just quoted, but could be any number, the two items are $x_{11}, x_{12}, x_{13}, \ldots, x_{1n}$ and $x_{21}, x_{22}, x_{23}, \ldots, x_{2n}$, and the distance between them is

$$d = \sqrt{[(x_{11}-x_{21})^2 + (x_{12}-x_{22})^2 + (x_{13}-x_{23})^2 + \ldots + (x_{1n}-x_{2n})^2]}$$

For a simple geometric example, the distance between two points in space, where one point has coordinates (1,2,1) and the other (2,2,4), the distance is

$$d = \sqrt{[(1-2)^2+(2-2)^2+(1-4)^2]}$$
$$d = \sqrt{[1+0+9]}$$
$$d = \sqrt{10}$$
$$d = 3.16 \text{ (to two decimal places)}$$

Non-hierarchical methods

In this form of clustering only one level of clusters is allowed, and the technique splits data into several clusters that do not overlap. Often you need to specify how many clusters you expect in the beginning. An example of non-hierarchical clustering is k-means clustering (see the example below).

Optimization techniques

These techniques are usually non-hierarchical. Again the number of groups is typically determined by the investigator and data are partitioned so as to optimize some predefined numerical measure (metric), as above. However, these techniques are typically iterative and involve large amounts of computing. Examples of optimization are unsupervised neural networks (e.g. Kohonen nets). Optimization is not necessarily going to produce a solution, and may give slightly different results on each run, and in some techniques the results can be totally different in some runs. Neural networks, for example, can get into 'local minima' and fail to reach a solution.

Density search techniques

In this technique cases are displayed on a graph, and areas of high density that are surrounded by more diffuse areas are considered to be clusters. This can be done by visual inspection.

Example: Hierarchical clustering

Using the Waterlow scores for 421 patients, of whom 69 went on to develop pressure sores, we would like to see how the Waterlow score splits patients into clusters, and if these clusters are those of patients with sores and patients with no sores.

In SPSS, selecting Statistics, then Classify, then Hierarchical Cluster will bring up a dialogue box shown in Figure 10.1, where we have entered the 11 variables of the Waterlow score (only six are shown, the rest would be visible using the scroll bar). By default, SPSS assumes that we want to cluster by cases (members). This may indeed be the case, and then we could look at the members of each cluster and interpret the meaning of the clusters. In the present example, clustering by cases would give such a large number of clusters (421) in the final stage of the analysis, that it would be very difficult to make much sense of it. Here we are better advised to see how the variables cluster, so we have elected to cluster by variable, which will give us at most 11 clusters (the original 11 variables).

SPSS gives a choice of plots: icicle plots (so named as they look like icicles hanging from the ceiling) or dendrograms. Figures 10.2 and 10.3 show such plots for the Waterlow data. The icicle plot starts with all the variables (or cases, if that option is selected) in the one cluster, this is row one. In the second row two clusters are formed, where the closest variables (or cases) are put into a cluster. In

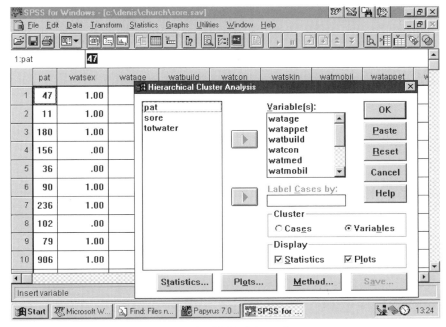

Figure 10.1   Hierarchical cluster analysis: SPSS dialogue box.

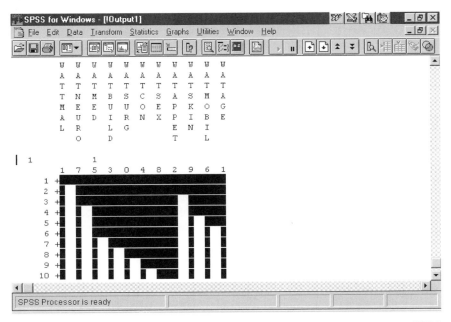

Figure 10.2   Waterlow scores for hospital patients clustered using an icicle diagram: SPSS Output screen.

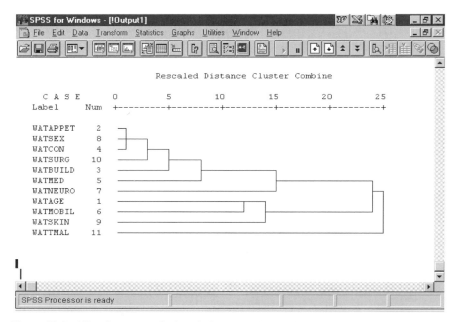

Figure 10.3 Waterlow scores for hospital patients clustered using a dendrogram: SPSS Output screen.

the present example it happens that one variable forms a cluster on its own (tissue malnourishment), with the other 10 forming the other cluster. 'The next row splits the data into three clusters: tissue malnutrition remains as one cluster, and the remaining ten variables split into two new clusters. Age mobility and skin are in one, and the remaining variables of the former 10-variable cluster of row one form the third cluster. This continues until there are ten clusters in the final row.'

I find the icicle plot difficult to follow, and prefer the dendrogram (Fig. 10.3). This can be read from right to left, in which case tissue malnourishment is the first variable to split off into a cluster, with all other variables in the other cluster. Then three clusters develop by the 10-variable cluster splitting into two: as above, age, mobility and skin form one, and the rest of the variables form the other cluster.

Reading the dendrogram the other way round, from left to right, appetite, gender and continence seem to be close together in on cluster, which then merges with surgery to form a slightly bigger cluster, etc.

There are several ways of interpreting this diagram (one of the difficulties of cluster analysis), but it seems to me that it could be seen conceptually as consisting of one cluster that is to do with general infirmity associated with age (and its consequences), shown by the cluster of age, mobility, skin and tissue malnutrition. The other (while not totally unrelated to age) appears to involve more extrinsic factors, such as recent surgery, medication and neurological deficit. Thus one cluster involves what happens to the patient, and the other describes the process of ageing. It is not clear to me, however, why gender is in the second cluster, other than it has to be in one of them, and I would have expected it to be in the age-related cluster (as there are more elderly women than men; indeed, a Mann–Whitney test does show a significant difference for this, $p < 0.05$).

Example: K-means clustering

This is a particularly useful technique when your data set is very large (over 200).[8] You must state the number of clusters that you think are appropriate, and the required number of clusters will be created. Using the Waterlow data again, we request two clusters. If the Waterlow score is inherently dividing subjects into sore and no sore groups, as we might hope, then the two clusters produced might be representative of a sore and a no sore cluster.

In SPSS the k-means cluster is obtained via the Statistics pull-down menu by selecting Classify then K-Means Cluster. The dialogue box will be similar to the one for hierarchical classification. If we click the Save option we can choose to save one or both derived variables, which are Cluster Membership and Distance From Cluster Centre. The former, which was selected, gives a new variable called QCL_1, which will contain the cluster number allocated to each case.

In the present example the k-means cluster analysis divided the data into the two clusters shown in Table 10.1. The values in brackets are the expected values obtained from a χ^2 calculation.

While a χ^2 analysis shows that it is most unlikely that the results would have occurred by chance ($p < 0.01$), i.e. that the variable 'sore' and the clustering variable are not independent, the correlation is not high, Cramer's V gives a value of 0.14. Thus the Waterlow score naturally splits into two clusters that are not very close to sore versus no sore groups. This does not mean that the Waterlow score does not help identify those patients who will go on to develop sores, but that the scoring scheme is capable of being split into different (although slightly correlated with eventual presence of a sore) clusters than presence or absence of sores.

Example: Infant, perinatal and neonatal mortality (hierarchical clustering)

A more meaningful (or at least easier to interpret) clustering is found in mortality figures. If we look at three measures of mortality for countries in Europe

Table 10.1 Clusters obtained from k-means cluster analysis of waterlow score data

	Cluster 1	Cluster 2
No sore	293 (284.3)	59 (67.7)
Sore	47 (55.7)	22 (13.3)

Values in parentheses are expected values (χ^2 calculation).

Table 10.2   Perinatal, neonatal and infant mortality around 1995 (data from WHO[13])

Country	Infant mortality	Perinatal mortality	Neonatal mortality rate
Albania	26	15	11
Moldova	25	30	15
Romania	23	15	10
Russian Federation	19	20	15
Belarus	17	15	10
Estonia	16	15	10
Ukraine	16	15	10
Hungary	15	10	10
Bulgaria	14	15	10
Latvia	14	20	10
Lithuania	13	15	10
Poland	13	20	15
Slovakia	12	15	10
Czech Republic	9	10	5
Greece	9	15	5
Portugal	9	10	5
France	7	10	6
Italy	7	10	5
Norway	7	5	5
Slovenia	7	10	5
Spain	7	5	5

(Table 10.2), infant mortality, perinatal mortality and neonatal mortality, we observe trends (some of the data from the smaller countries have been removed for clarity, but the overall picture is not altered by this). However, the three measures are not in the same rank order for all values. For example, Albania has the worst infant mortality, but Moldova has the worst perinatal mortality and Albania the fifth worst. We could use all three measures together to see which countries cluster together (Fig. 10.4).

Working from the right to the left of the dendrogram shown in the figure, Moldova appears as a cluster on its own. It has, in general, the worst figures of all, although not on every measure, as noted above. The dendrogram splits into two, with an almost complete split into western European and eastern Europe. In the eastern countries, Russia, Poland and Latvia cluster closely, and most of the former state-socialist countries that were outside the borders of the USSR (Slovakia, Lithuania, Estonia, etc.) are also close to each other. You will note that the western countries have very few levels, and are thus much more similar to each other than are the eastern countries. The only former state-socialist countries that are in the western cluster are Slovenia and the Czech Republic. These data can be interpreted as a massive difference between eastern and western Europe with respect to infant, perinatal and neonatal mortality, but with much more diversity in the east. Note that the clustering algorithm had no information on the geography of the countries, merely the mortality data.

Further interpretation is possible given extra information, For example, the two former state-socialist countries (Slovenia and the Czech Republic) were among the

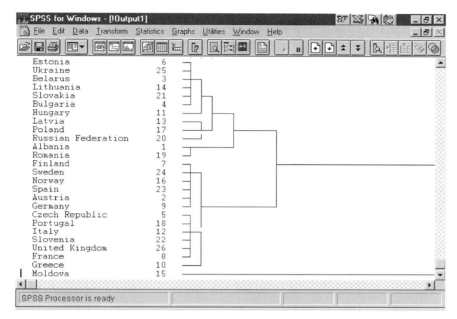

Figure 10.4   Morality data for European countries clustered using a dendrogram: SPSS Output screen.

richer of the former eastern bloc countries. They also had much more liberal economic policies, and therefore would have less difficulty adjusting to the post-Communist transition, and they are geographically close to rich western countries (e.g. Austria and Germany) with whom they could more easily trade. As stated above, the smaller countries, such as Iceland, which were removed to make the data more manageable for the displays fall into the clusters that one might expect, e.g. Iceland clusters with other wealthy western countries.

Problems with cluster analysis

Optimization techniques typically require large amounts of computing time, and in the case of neural networks scale badly, are not guaranteed to give a solution, and any solution found may be difficult to analyse.

It is difficult to choose the optimal metric in hierarchical clustering, the solution is sensitive to the chosen metric, and the clustering may be difficult to interpret.

DISCRIMINANT ANALYSIS

Suppose we wish to identify patients who will develop some condition, and have data that consist of several variables. The task is, given the data, to classify patients into two (or more) groups. Discriminant analysis is a technique that addresses this problem. It is a linear technique, and is based on Bayesian analysis. In discriminant analysis a value is returned by some linear combination of the variables which, it is hoped, will distinguish between the two (or more) groups.

Bayes' theorem[9,10] gives the probability of being in a group, given additional information. The theorem is expressed as[10]

$$P(G_i \mid D) = \frac{P(D \mid G_i)P(G_i)}{\sum_{i=1}^{n} P(D \mid G_i)P(G_i)}$$

where: G_i is group i (i = 1, 2, 3, etc.); D is the value of the discriminant function; $P(G_i)$ is the probability that a case (a patient in our example) is in group i, where no other information is available and is termed the *prior probability*; $P(D|G_i)$ is the probability of getting a given discriminant function value if a case is in a given group, and is termed the *conditional probability*; and $P(G_i|D)$ is the probability that a case is in group i given a discriminant function D.

Let us now revisit the Waterlow score data used in other chapters (e.g. Chs 8 and 11). The problem here can be stated that we wish to work out which of two groups (sore versus non-sore) the patient is in, given the eleven sub-scores of the Waterlow score.

In the real world we have computed D, and want to get $P(G_i|D)$. SPSS performs the computations via the Statistics pull-down menu, from which you select Classify and then Discriminant. A dialogue box then requires a grouping variable to be used, and you need to enter the range of values that will form the required groups. In the present case a variable called 'sore' is either 0 or 1, so the range contains just those two numbers. Next, the (one or more) independent variables are entered, which here are the 11 subscores.

By default, SPSS ascribes equal prior probabilities to all groups, so in our case of two groups it would allocate 50% probability to getting a sore and 50% to not getting a sore. But in our example this allocation of probability is not appropriate, as there are far more patients without sores than patients with sores, so it is better to get SPSS to use the proportions of groups found in the data as prior probabilities, which are about 83% for no sores and 17% for sores. This option is selected from the Classify option in the Discriminant dialogue box.

The Discriminant procedure can give standardized or unstandardized coefficients for the discriminant function. Unstandardized coefficients apply directly to the raw variables, but are sensitive to the scales used. Thus a high coefficient does not imply that the variable is more important than another one with a lower coefficient. Standardization is therefore typically used in order to show better the relative importance of variables.

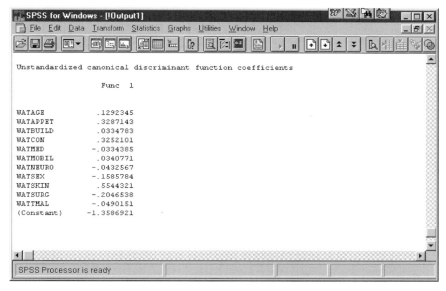

Figure 10.5   Discriminant analysis: SPSS Output screen.

The output is an equation, the *discriminant equation*, obtained from the unstandardized coefficients, as shown in Figure 10.5. The equation is, therefore,

$$D = (\text{WATAGE} \times 0.1292345) + (\text{WATAPPET} \times 0.3287143)$$
$$+ (\text{WATBUILD} \times 0.0334783) + (\text{WATCON} \times 0.3252101)$$
$$- (\text{WATMED} \times 0.0334385) + (\text{WATMOBIL} \times 0.0340771)$$
$$- (\text{WATNEURO} \times 0.0432567) - (\text{WATSEX} \times 0.1585784)$$
$$+ (\text{WATSKIN} \times 0.5544321) - (\text{WATSURG} \times 0.2046538)$$
$$- (\text{WATTMAL} \times 0.0490151) - 1.3586921$$

This equation is used to compute the probability of a case belonging to one or other of the groups. This probability can be saved via the Save option in the dialogue box. ROC analysis (see Ch. 8) may be used to check the ability of the classification of the discriminant function. In an ROC, plot sensitivity and (1 – specificity) are plotted for a variety of thresholds, which here could be the probability values obtained from the discriminant analysis. The area under the curve obtained indicates the accuracy of the classification. A random classification would contain half the area, i.e. a diagonal line from bottom left to top right; a perfect plot would be as far from the diagonal as possible. An ROC plot was done for the Waterlow score (see Fig. 10.6), where the plot is seen to be much better than random.

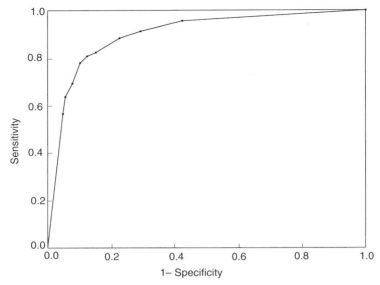

Figure 10.6   A ROC plot of the discriminant analysis of Waterlow scores.

In general, discriminant analysis is used as an exploratory technique to identify possible causative variables. The assumptions of discriminant analysis include normality of the independent variables, and that the relationships are inherently linear. According to the SPSS advanced user's guide,[11] it is not rigorously correct to use a dependent variable that is an event that either occurs or does not occur, and the example discussed above is just such a case. However, as the technique is typically used in an exploratory way, the assumptions may be relaxed provided you do not use the results in a strictly inferential manner. Given that the example shown in the SPSS guide is survival or death in infants with respiratory distress syndrome,[12] such a use as above may be considered acceptable. However, logistic regression, which makes fewer assumptions, is designed for use in binary dependent variables and gives a probability of occurrence of an event occurring, may be preferred (see Ch. 6).

CONCLUSION

If you wish to explore data to generate theories based on possible relationships among data, either with respect to individuals or variables, cluster analysis is a potential choice of technique. It will produce either simple (non-hierarchical) clusters or clusters in several levels with complex relationships (hierarchical).

If you already have the groupings of interest, and want to predict which group an individual is in given some set of variables, then discriminant analysis is a technique to consider.

EXERCISES

1. Look at the cluster dendrogram below for mortality of men aged 20–24 years (inclusive). To which group of countries (CEE, EU or former USSR) does the Czech Republic appear to belong? In terms of young male mortality, is Latvia closer to the Ukraine or Poland?

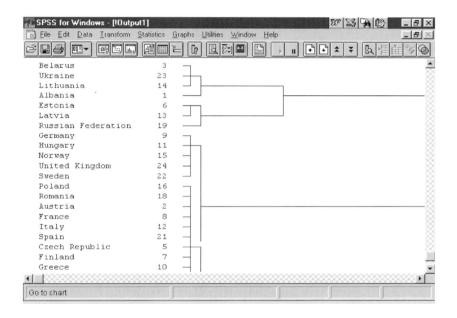

2. Using gross domestic product (GDP) and infant, perinatal and neonatal mortality for 25 countries, the three country types (CEE = 1, EU = 2 and former USSR = 3) were used in a discriminant analysis. The output is shown below. Using function 1, determine to which group the following rates (for Belarus) apply:

GDP	Infant	Perinatal	Neonatal
1500.00	17.00	15.00	10.00

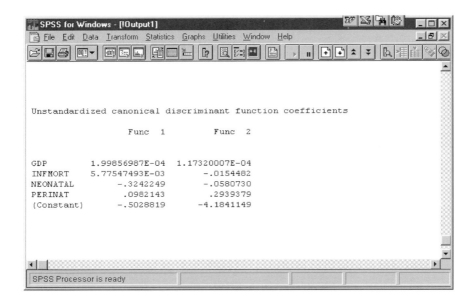

REFERENCES

1. Everitt B 1980 Cluster analysis. Heinemann, London
2. Lachenbruch P A 1975 Discriminant analysis. Macmillan, New York
3. Cooley W W, Lohnes P P 1971 Multivariate data analysis. Wiley, New York
4. Gorsuch R L 1974 Factor analysis. W B Saunders, Philadelphia
5. Manly B F J 1986 Multivariate statistical analysis. Chapman & Hall, London
6. Hammond S 1995 Introduction to multivariate data analysis. In: Brakwell G M, Hammond S, Fife-Schaw C (eds) Research methods in psychology. Sage, London, p 360–385
7. Norusis M J 1994 SPSS professional statistics 6.1. SPSS, Chicago, IL, p 127–142
8. Norusis M J 1994 SPSS professional statistics 6.1. SPSS, Chicago, IL, p 111
9. Mosteller F, Rourke R, Thomas G 1970 Probability with statistical applications, 2nd edn. Addison-Wesley, London, p 158–164
10. Norusis M J 1994 SPSS professional statistics 6.1. SPSS, Chicago, IL, p 9
11. Norusis M J 1990 SPSS advanced statistics user's guide. SPSS, Chicago, IL, p 45
12. Norusis M J 1990 SPSS advanced statistics user's guide. SPSS, Chicago, IL, p 1–43
13. WHO 1996 Perinatal mortality. World Health Organization, Geneva

11

Neural networks and genetic algorithms

Computers are very good at performing complex calculations; something humans find difficult. However, computers are very poor at many tasks we find very straightforward, for example recognizing faces, or interpreting speech. This has led some scientists to create new computer programs that try to mimic the way a brain functions, to achieve tasks such as speech recognition. These have also been very useful in medical applications such as EEG and ECG (EKG in the USA) recognition.

Other workers have noted that biological systems evolve rather than are designed, and have simulated evolution to improve computer programs. This has also led to medical applications such as gait analysis.

KEY POINTS

- Neural networks and genetic algorithms are optimizing methods
- In a neural network or genetic algorithm the solution is not guaranteed, or necessarily repeatable
- Neural networks and genetic algorithms 'learn' a solution, rather than adopting a rule-based approach
- Neural networks and genetic algorithms can solve non-linear problems
- If the problem is inherently linear, then traditional statistical methods are preferred to neural networks.

At the end of this chapter the student should be able to:

1. *List the advantages and disadvantages of employing a neural network or genetic algorithm approach*

2. *Understand when a neural network or genetic algorithm solution may be useful.*

3. *State some of the possible techniques for making a solution by neural networks more plausible*

INTRODUCTION

Most of the chapters in this book have concentrated on specific statistical techniques commonly used in health research, and available as modules in, or at least computable (in principle) using SPSS. This chapter is an exception. Neural networks are beyond the capabilities of SPSS in its current form, and other packages need to be considered. Neural network packages are available as commercial products, such as Neural Ware, or as shareware or public domain (i.e. typically free for non-commercial use), such as the PDP, PlaNet and Genesis packages. A package that is free and available for IBM compatible PCs and most other platforms is NevProp (I used version 3.0 for the examples in this chapter).[1] Some mathematical packages can be modified to create neural networks, or have modules for neural computing (e.g. matlab). I do not try to show you how to implement neural networks, but rather to introduce you to this topic. Thus a more discursive treatment of the subject is given, with applications in medicine and related areas noted.

All the statistical methods used so far in this book have been based on algorithms, or a series of steps that can be codified into a formula, which can be solved by a calculator, either human or electronic. Computers have speeded up these types of calculation, so that tests that might take days to compute by hand can be done in seconds or less. With these mathematical problems, computers are very much better at achieving a solution (more accurate, more reliable, much faster).

Computer programs are typically sequential (i.e. they do one thing at a time), but because each step is completed very quickly the solution is achieved in a short space of time. The program is based around an algorithm, or a series of steps. For example, to work out the dose of a drug for an infant, the algorithm might be:

1. Measure the baby's weight

2. Multiply the weight by some (constant) number
3. Give the drug.

This is a very simple algorithm, but if you had to compute the drug dosages for all possible infant weights, to produce a reference table for example, it would take you a long time. It would be much better to use a computer to produce the table, which it could do within a second or two.

However, certain types of problem are not amenable to solution by a typical mathematical approach, and standard computer programs have not been very successful in solving them. But these are precisely the problems that humans find quite straightforward, taking split seconds to solve in some cases. Consider the following two examples:

- *Image recognition.* We can see and recognize an object that is rotated, partially obscured, in poor light, and either enlarged or reduced in size. Devising computer programs to do this is possible but very difficult. The programs tend to be very specific, e.g. enabling a robot to locate an identical piece of machinery whichever way round it is presented to it. Writing very general programs that allow a vision system to recognize anything in its view is extremely difficult, if not impossible, using conventional programming techniques.
- *NP complete problems.* These form a class of problems that scale badly.[2,3] The solutions are typically easy to formulate, but become massively increasingly time consuming to work out. That is, they may be simple to work out in principle, and take a small amount of time to work out for small problems, but the time taken increases exponentially as the problem gets bigger. The classic example is the travelling salesman problem. A salesman needs to visit several cities, and wants to know the most efficient (shortest in time or distance) way to arrange his itinerary. It is simple to state the solution: work out all possible paths and choose the shortest. It is fast to compute the routes for three or four cities, but as the number of cities increases it becomes impossible to work out every possible path. The computation is related to the *factorial* of the number of cities. If the number of cities is n, then the computation is $n!$ (read n factorial), which is $n(n-1)(n-2)$, ..., 1. So for $n = 5$ the number of possible paths would be $5 \times 4 \times 3 \times 2 \times 1$. Even on a fast supercomputer, it can take millions of years to compute the number of paths for even a relatively small number of cities. It appears counterintuitive that such simply formulated problems cannot be solved simply by adding computer power. However, if a single calculation between two cities takes 1 ns (one-thousandth of one-millionth of a second), then for 10 cities it will take about 0.004 s, for 11 cities about 0.04 s, for 13 cities 6.2 s, for fifteen cities 22 minutes, for 16 cities nearly 6 h, for 17 cities over 4 days, for 19 cities nearly 4 years, 20 cities over 77 years, and 22 cities over 35 000 years!

NP-complete problems

An NP-complete problem is one that has three main features. It is simple to define the problem; it is easy to solve the problem when the problem is small; but it very quickly becomes impossible to solve, even in principle, as the problem grows in size. The classic NP-complete problem is the 'travelling salesman problem', whereby you need to visit several cities and want to work out the shortest route. This is easy to define (find the shortest route for several cities), easy to solve for three or four cities, but very difficult to solve for even a small number (try 10 yourself!).

Why is the NP complete problem so difficult? If there are two cities, starting at one city, there are two paths, from city A to city B, and vice versa, i.e. one distance, no problem. For three cities there are six paths; starting at A, you can choose to go on either of two paths, having chosen one, there is only one path left. But you could have started at any of the three cities, and therefore the total number of paths is 3×2. If there were four cities, then having chosen a particular city (say A) there are now three cities left, which is the problem we have already worked out (3×2), but again we could have started at any of the four cities, so the total number of solutions is 4×3×2 (or 4!). Adding each new city adds a new term to the formula for the total number of paths, so for five cities it is 5×4×3×2 (or 5!). So adding a city to give not four but five cities does not make the problem 25% more difficult, but 500% more difficult, and each new city makes the problem increasingly worse, adding a tenth city makes the problem 10 times harder than for nine cities, but the nine-city problem is nine times worse than the eight-city problem, and so on. The 10-city problem is 9000% more complex than the eight-city problem, although only 25% more cities have been added. This is what we mean by scaling badly.

The obvious thing to note is that, while a computer cannot work out, for example, the travelling salesman problem, the salesman does not take several million years to work out an itinerary, but manages to produce a workable solution within a few minutes. So some problems can be solved by humans easily and quickly, yet are not amenable to solution by massive computers. How does the salesman perform this apparent miracle? Features of the human solution are:

- The salesman does not calculate the solution exactly, if he did he would be acting like a computer, and would take even longer. He accepts a solution that is good enough, i.e. he looks for a few solutions, and takes one that is sufficiently speedy that there is no point looking further. Clearly, if doing the visits for 20 cities takes a week, then spending an hour planning it may make sense if it cuts down the overall trip by a few hours. Equally, there is no point spending several days on the problem to reduce the trip by another hour or two. The salesman is pragmatic, and takes an acceptable, but suboptimal solution.

- The salesman does not even look at certain possibilities. For example, if there were two cities A and B a few miles apart, going from one of these, say city A, to a very distant city (city C), then back to city B, would not normally be considered, as it is clearly very inefficient. Thus the problem is reduced by only looking at part of the solutions possible.
- The salesman has done these trips before. He has experience and recognizes certain paths as better than others without working them out, in fact the real salesman probably never works the distances out, but even if he did when he started to do the job, after a while he probably does not need to. He relies on recognition from previous similar solutions. He may not have done exactly the same set of cities in one tour, but he has done sufficiently similar ones that his experience works for him.

A parallel exists in a common problem encountered in nursing, that of rostering. If one has three members of staff, covering (say) two shifts with weekends, etc., such that on any given day two staff work on opposite shifts, this is a simple problem to work out. As there are only so many possibilities, each one could all be tried. However, you might have 30 staff working on a ward. You can see that having selected one staff member for a shift there are 29 left, so the problem is now smaller, but you could have selected any of the members of staff first, so there are 30 such initial problems. Having got the smaller 29-staff problem, you can now select any of the 29 staff next, leaving the smaller 28 staff rostering problem; but there are 29 such solutions. In fact the problem is worse as you must have a certain staff mix, and you may know staff nurses A and B hate each other, and will not work well together, and then someone goes sick so you need to recalculate the rosta. The ward sister hates doing the rosta, but, without a computer she can usually manage to do a reasonable job. It is clear from the foregoing that a computer will not necessarily help her if it looks exhaustively at every possible permutation of staff. What she needs is a computer program that works like she does. It should learn from experience and, when working out the rosta, should stop when a reasonable solution is found, and not look for the ideal, as that would take several centuries or more.

ARTIFICIAL NEURAL NETWORKS

Such a type of solution is possible using programs that try to mimic how we think. These are called artificial neural networks (ANNs). The original idea is almost as old as modern computing itself. For example, Hebb[4] produced an ANN algorithm in the late 1940s. The idea is to use the same architecture that the brain uses to solve the problem. Computers work *sequentially* – an algorithm is a series of steps, calculated one after the other very quickly (thousandths or millionths of a second). This works fine for accounting problems, solving complex equations in space travel, or performing statistical analysis, i.e. for the functions that we tend to use computers for. But it is not the way the brain works. The brain is parallel, and works slowly (each operation takes of the order of hundredths or tenths of a second or more). But the brain does certain things better, as illustrated above. So perhaps we can improve computer programs for certain tasks by working with parallel programs, where several calculations are worked out simultaneously.

Simulated annealing

One such ANN solution was proposed by analogy with a physical observation. If a metal is cooled down slowly it makes much better crystals than if it is cooled down quickly. The molecules can arrange themselves into a crystal structure when they are at a certain temperature; cooling the molecules down freezes them into place. If the molecules are not in a good crystal formation and are cooled too quickly they have too little energy (heat) to move again and are stuck in a suboptimal crystal, but if cooled slowly they can get out of poor structures and form more perfect structures before being frozen. The physical explanation for this phenomena is that the more organized crystal structure takes more energy to break than a less good one. The higher the temperature the faster the molecules are moving, i.e. the more the energy they have, on average. But some molecules will have more energy than others, so at a given temperature there is a possibility of breaking up a crystal structure that has formed. However, this is more likely to happen to poor crystal structures, and gets less likely as the temperature lowers. Lowering the temperature rapidly leaves much of the crystal in its first attempt at ordering, which is likely to be poor. Slow lowering of the temperature allows most of these poor structure to be replaced by better ones, which are themselves less likely to break up. Making good metal crystals by slow cooling is called annealing.

This idea could be applied to the travelling salesman problem, whereby the distance (or time) between cities could be considered analogous to the energy, and starting at a totally random position (i.e. almost certainly very poor) at any given moment there could be a possibility of replacing each path with another. The possibility of changing can be called the temperature. High temperature connections with low energy can be broken, but are less likely to be replaced than high energy connections. As the temperature is lowered it is increasingly unlikely that low energy connections will be replaced. So, slowly reducing the temperature should allow poor solutions to be replaced by better ones. Such an algorithm that mimics the slow cooling of metals is called simulated annealing. It is important to realize that simulated annealing is only a model – there is no temperature, no energy and there are no crystals forming. However, the algorithm treats the possibility of replacing a path *as if* it were a slowly cooling temperature, i.e. it reduces slowly from very likely (hot) to quite possible (warm) to very unlikely (cold) over time; and the distance or time between cities is likened to energy, in that the smaller the value the more energy it is said to possess, making it more difficult (but always possible) to change.

This algorithm has several interesting parallels with the human solution:

- It is not guaranteed to be perfect, in fact it almost certainly will not be. But it tends to get better the longer the algorithm takes to run.
- At any given time in the algorithm a solution can be replaced with a worse one, but overall it tends to improve over time.
- The algorithm has an end-point that can be determined, you can say 'Give me a solution in an hour' for example. The time taken to run the algorithm can depend on the cost of running it.
- It is a parallel problem. Each of the paths can be changing at the same time, so where you go from city A can be calculated separately from where you go after city B.
- It is possible to visit one city more than once, which seems inefficient, but if the solution is better than the ones found so far you may accept that.

Simulated annealing has been described[5,6] where the algorithm may be run several times, and the best solution chosen. This may be necessary as the algorithm can result in a severely suboptimal solution, a so-called *local minimum*. Look at Figure 11.1. Suppose this represents the energy (distance or time in the travelling salesman problem), so that a low value is better than a high value. The minimum we can reach on this curve is the best we

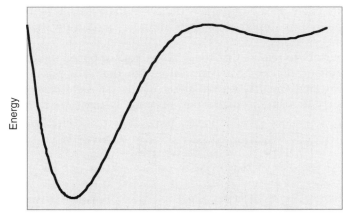

Time

Figure 11.1 Illustration of the local minimum problem.

can do. If you start at the left, then the solution falls into the left-hand (and much lower) minimum. But if you start at the right, the solution could get stuck in an energy state not much better than the start of the problem, and fails to get into the neighbouring solution. Imagine rolling a ball down the slope, given enough initial speed it might jump over the bump to land in the lower (better) minimum, but given a lower starting speed it might fall in the worse (right-hand, higher) solution.

The Boltzmann machine is one algorithm for producing simulated annealing, and may be solved using a sequential method, but can also be solved in a parallel fashion by using an ANN.

Auto-associative ANNs

The Boltzmann machine when implemented in an ANN, is one of a type known as an auto-associative ANN. These networks produce input and output using the same units, or neurons. There are many types, such as the Brain State in a Box[7] and Hopfield Nets.[8] Consider Figure 11.2. The boxes represent the artificial neurons (usually called units), and the artificial axons (usually called links) are represented by arrows (you can think of the links ending in artificial synapses to artificial dendrites; however, in ANN work these are typically ignored). Each link has a weight, which you may see as analogous to the rate of firing of a real neuron; the weight is the strength of the link between two units. If this was a representation of the travelling salesman problem, cities could be modelled as neurons, and the likelihood of going from one city to another could be the value carried on the axon. An auto-associative network is so called because the inputs and outputs are the same. In the salesman problem the input is the initial (random) paths, and the output is an improved (hopefully) set of paths between the cities. In a computer simulation the artificial neurons (units) and artificial axons (links) are simply numbers stored on the computer's memory or disk store.

It is important to realize that the ANN is not supposed to be an accurate or even realistic model of a brain, although that is a possible research direction. Rather, the ANN uses some of the characteristics of nervous systems to try to solve problems that nervous systems are rather good at.

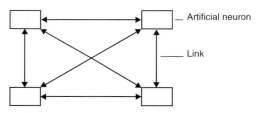

Figure 11.2 An auto-associative network.

In particular, the mathematics used in ANNs is almost certainly nothing like what goes on in real nervous systems, and the complexity of real nervous systems is orders of magnitude higher than that of ANNs. However, ANNs are not required to perform all the tasks of a real nervous system or brain, but to solve discrete, well-defined problems. They may in time be comparable in complexity and performance to subsystems of the brain, and may be similar in operation, but not yet.

Hetero-associative ANNs

Brains are highly connected. The retina alone has roughly 100 000 000 neurons, each connected to between hundreds to hundreds of thousands of others.[9] Even if there are only hundreds of connections for all neurons, this gives the order of 10 billion or more connections. There is a great deal of information that can be 'hard wired' with the number of neurons in the cerebral hemispheres and the massive connectivity. It is plausible that the reason why humans and other animals can react quickly with (by electronic standards) very slow brains is that they have learned reactions, which are encoded in the connections of the brain. Thus highly connected parallel computing machines that are trained are an attractive proposition.

Auto-associative ANNs can be seen as methods of 'cleaning up' an input. For example, an image that is incomplete or rotated could be translated into a similar but corrected image. However, in many problems you want to classify data into different categories. An example of this type of problem is the visual recognition problem. A potentially infinite number of views of animals needs to be classified into those that are dogs, those that are cats, etc., or into images of ships that are on our side or the enemy side. In health care it might be the problem of classifying all the bacterial plates containing *Escherichia coli* from those containing some other organism, or of those mammograms that show normal breasts from those that are potentially cancerous, or those radiographs that show a fracture from those that do not.

All these visual recognition problems have some common characteristics.

• The input is a data source composed of the light intensity at many points (we will ignore colour for the sake of simplicity).
• The output is the classification of the input into two or more categories.
• The output is not necessarily or usually of the same number of dimensions as the input. For example, if the image of a mammogram containing 16 pixels by 32 pixels were used you would have 512 inputs, but if the interpretation of the image could be either 'normal' or 'malignant', there could be two outputs, one for each diagnosis. In fact one output would do,

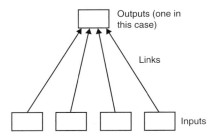

Figure 11.3 A hetero-associative network.

as we could say the output was 0 for normal and 1 for malignant, for example.

Such networks where the inputs and outputs are not the same are called hetero-associative, as you are attempting to associate two different things, in the above case an image with a diagnosis. Such a network is shown as in Figure 11.3. Note that the links here are one way, going from inputs to outputs only, and not back again. In ANNs the output units are typically considered to be switched on or off. This could be achieved by outputting a number in the range 0.0–1.0, where a value below 0.1 indicates switched off, a value above 0.9 indicates switched on, and other values indicate either on or off. Alternatively, the output could be seen as a percentage risk or likelihood, so 0.1 means 10% risk, 0.2 means 20% risk, etc. In the network shown in Figure 11.3 four inputs are linked to just one output. This might be four risk factors for decubitus ulcer as inputs with an output that is turned on for high risk, and turned off for low risk, or it could be four parameters from an electrocardiogram (ECG) reading, the output being the presence or absence of some disease, for example myocardial infarct.

Such networks were devised in the late 1940s by Rosenblatt,[10] who called them perceptrons. The strength of a link is called its weight, and takes a numerical value. The inputs and outputs are also numbers. The perceptron works by weighting and summing each input to give an output. This is achieved by multiplying the weight between the input unit and output unit by the input value for each input, and the sum of these is the output:

Output = Σ weight of link × Value of input

The network can 'learn'. This is achieved by presenting to the network data for which we have a known classification. We might, for example, give an ECG reading and state that it is one from a diseased heart, and then give another ECG that is normal. The weights are then altered to reduce the difference between the target (what it should be) and the output (what it actually is). An iterative approach is taken, the weights being updated after each pattern until the error reduces to a minimum. The details are not given here, but may be found in Rumelhart et al.[7]

It has been shown by Minsky & Papert[11,12] that these networks are capable of solving any problem for which a linear solution exists, but equally some very simple non-linear problems are completely incapable of solution, even in principle, by such networks. Unfortunately, one of these problems is related to identifying connectedness in space, i.e. whether two parts of the visual field are part of the same object or not. Humans can clearly do this, so a perceptron, whatever else it may be able to do, can certainly not provide the model for human visual cognitive ability. After Minsky & Papert's book, research on ANNs almost ground to a halt, as it appeared that it was not possible to solve many of the problems that interested cognitive scientists (for example), and linear problems are very easily solved using standard statistical techniques such as regression, as shown in other chapters of this book.

In 1986, Rumelhart & McClelland[13] showed that perceptrons could solve non-linear problems if an extra layer of units was placed between the input and output units, so called 'hidden' units (because their value is not defined by the programmer, but arise in the course of the network solving the problem). The perceptrons with hidden layers are called *multi-layer perceptrons* (MLPs) (Fig. 11.4).

Learning in MLPs

An MLP learns by being given examples, i.e. it is trained, or 'supervised' (in contradistinction to auto-associative networks, which tend to organize themselves without external training). Initially, a set of inputs (a pattern) is presented to the network by setting the input units to appropriate values. The network, starting initially from a random set of link weights,

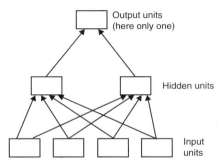

Figure 11.4 A multi-layer perceptron (MLP).

gives its output, which is likely to be totally incorrect. The difference between the output of the network and what it should have given (the target) is the error. If the target and the output are very close, the difference is very small. If the network weights are altered in proportion to this difference (i.e. more for large differences), the network will hopefully settle down to a solution that is reasonably accurate. Thus the error is used to adjust the weights in order to improve the output. Then a new input pattern is given. The process continues until all training patterns have been completed, and then the entire set is shown to the network again (there are theoretical reasons for showing all patterns first and then updating the weights, and this is often done in practice). This is repeated until the network settles down to some solution. The trick is to find some way of changing the weights to improve the outputs based on the difference between the output and the value the network should give.

But for the MLP the situation is a bit more complicated. The error is propagated back from the output, through the hidden layer, and used to adjust the weights between the output and the hidden unit, and between the hidden unit and the input layers. However, in principle, the situation is similar to the simple perceptron case. Because the error is propagated back through the network, these MLPs are often called *back-propagation networks*. Details of the mathematics involved in changing the weights of an MLP to reduce the error can be found in Rumelhart et al.[7]

Uses of ANNs in health research

There are a number of papers describing the use of ANNs in medical and medical physics applications, but (to my knowledge) none describing their use in nursing, physiotherapy or other professions allied to medicine (PAM). However, some of the problems in nursing and PAM would seem to be tractable with an ANN approach. A summary of medical imaging applications of ANNs is given by Anthony.[14]

When the rules are not known

Suppose you want to build an expert system, i.e. a (usually computer based) system that emulates an expert. You will need to spend a lot of time with an expert finding out the rules. However, in some cases the expert *recognizes* a situation (say a diagnosis) but cannot tell you why. As the expert in these cases typically learned from experience, possibly you can get an ANN to do the same.

An expert system may be built by imputing numerical values representing knowledge items into the input layer of an ANN. Indeed one of the most commonly documented medical applications of ANNs is the manufacture of expert systems. Chest pain (for example) has been used to classify high, medium and low risk cardiac patients.[15] In a comparison with a symbolic expert system that was designed to diagnose headaches, an MLP has been built which took as inputs numeric coded answers to 216 questions into 216 input units.[16] In addition to answers to medical history questions, laboratory test results and ECG (EKG in the USA) findings have been input into an MLP designed to diagnose acute myocardial infarction (heart attack).[17] A similar expert system using MLPs has been constructed to diagnose carcinoma of the lung.[18]

Impedance imaging. By applying a small current to two electrodes, and using the output voltages from an array of electrodes surrounding an organ or limb, etc., it is possible to reconstruct an image. There are difficulties with the reconstruction techniques, however, and many simplifying assumptions are used. MLPs have been used[19] to solve the inverse problem; i.e. given the voltages, the conductivity distribution that would have caused such outputs is determined.

Pattern matching

Image processing is a classic pattern matching problem. For example, tumour staging may be accomplished by the use of thermal imaging. Seven stages of tumour were identified in a study using white mice.[20] Taking the pixels from a thermal image as input to an ANN, it was possible to classify the tumours.

In medical applications, diagnosis from the ECG and electroencephalogram (EEG) is another pattern matching problem.

ECG pattern recognition. Applications for ECG include the following:

- The detection of abnormal ECGs. A bi-directional associative memory (a type of auto-associate network) model was used to detect abnormal ECG patterns.[21] This is an easier problem than classifying ECGs. Abnormal ECGs were detected with less than 1% error.
- Back-propagation has been used to classify ECG signals based on five parameters extracted from the ECG reading.[22]
- Classification of arrhythmias has been achieved using an auto-associative model.[23] The net distinguished between normal QRS and arrhythmias with high accuracy. Classification of ECGs using five features extracted from the readings and used as input to an MLP has been used to place the ECGs into six diagnostic classes.[23]

EEG pattern recognition. Electroencephalographic data have been analysed using back-propagation ANNs to identify spikes.[24] In preliminary experiments on test data the ANN was able to identify the spikes with high precision. EEG patterns are difficult to classify due to their noise and complexity.[25] Typical EEG studies use external stimuli to provoke an EEG reaction. Hiraiwa et al[25] have used the readiness potential, the EEG pattern produced just prior to voluntary muscle movement, to train an ANN. The muscle movements were those produced when the subject pronounced syllables. The ANN was able to distinguish correctly 16 of 30 new patterns as belonging to one of five syllable groups.

Nuclear medicine. MLPs have been used to differentiate between normal and abnormal thallium-201 scintigrams which can be used to show coronary artery disease. Three parameters were computed for each of five segments of three views, and these 45 values were fed into an MLP.[26] Test data gave an accuracy of 82% for diagnosing cardiac disease. Pulmonary scintigrams have been classified with very limited success using back-propagation on the principal components (see Ch. 9) of images.[27]

Nuclear magnetic resonance (NMR). Back-propagation has been employed[28] to segment NMR into seven distinct tissue types (background, fat and skin, stroke, ventricle, cerebrospinal fluid, grey matter, and white matter). An ANN took the pixels as input, one at a time, and learnt to which class the pixels belonged, i.e. to which tissue type.

Grossberg & Mingolla[29] have developed neural models of vision systems that have been used to process NMR images. It was concluded that the ANN extracted the invariant features needed for pattern recognition.

Radiography. Very little work has been undertaken in the area of radiological applications of ANNs. A simulation study has shown some potential efficacy in this area.[31] A synthetic nodule was created by placing a 3 pixel by 3 pixel square centrally in a 5 pixel by 5 pixel grid. Pseudo-Gaussian noise was added, and a network trained with a set of images, half of which contained a nodule. Receiver operating curves (see Ch. 8) were plotted for test (unseen) images with a variety of signal to noise ratios (SNRs). The training set had an SNR of 15.0, and test sets with SNR values of 1.5 and 3.0 were used. In comparison to human observers, who had been trained to distinguish the nodules, the ANN outperformed the human observers for both SNRs. It was concluded that the ANN could detect signals with better performance than human observers. However, it is noted that the signals were very simple, and not representative of clinical radiographs.[32]

Drug therapy. An MLP has been used to estimate the pharmacokinetic properties of drugs. A comparison was made between the MLP, the maximum likelihood (ML) estimation and the maximum a posteriori probability (MAP). The MLP performed well in estimating the distribution volume and elimination clearance of theophylline.[33,34]

Mammograms. Work has been done[35] to remove irrelevant detail from mammograms using ANNs. The mammogram image has a background and textural information, etc., which is easily ignored by a human operator, to allow attention to be focused on the area of the image containing the clinical detail. An ANN was explored to determine its effectiveness in emulating the human factor. A similar technique was described by Anthony and co-workers,[27,36] where segments extracted from a nuclear image, some of which contained lung fields and some of which were artefacts, were classified by an MLP. The MLP was able to classify correctly 'unseen' (i.e. not presented to the network in training) segments so that a subsequent net could be used to accept only segments of interest.

Image reconstruction

Ultrasound. Ultrasound is used as an imaging modality. There have been attempts to produce tomographic images, in a similar fashion as in X-ray, NMR and nuclear studies. However, there are problems associated with the relatively large wavelength (diffraction and refraction effects) and anisotropy (different properties of the material in different directions). Tomogram reconstruction techniques often use simplifying assumptions in order to avoid considering these effects. ANNs were used to solve the inverse problem; i.e. given the times of flight (or amplitude, or some other attribute) of the ultrasound beam through a specimen, the structure that would produce the data was deduced.[37] While this is geared to non-destructive testing of materials, the relevance to medical imaging is obvious. Previous work has been undertaken in which an MLP was trained with the transducer pressures obtained using a range of cylindrical objects as test specimens. The ANN was able to learn the size of the scanned object from the projection data.[38] Holographic images have been created using ultrasound rays, where a three-layer MLP learned to output images of letters of the alphabet.[39] The wave velocity within a tissue is usually considered to be constant, but may vary by up to 8%.[40] An MLP with two hidden layers was used to correct the delay noise that occurred as a result of the assumption of constant velocity. A substantial improvement was obtained in simulations.

Problems and difficulties with the ANN methods

Performance

An ANN is not necessarily going to out-perform other algorithms, nor is it even guaranteed to produce any sort of solution. In almost all, if not all cases, it is a matter of faith whether the neural network will give improved results.

Consider, for example, the diagnosis of headaches.[16] The symbolic expert system performed slightly better (accuracy 70%) than the MLP (accuracy 67%) for a test set of 94 patients. However, an MLP for ECG interpretation gave a detection rate of 92% and false-positive rate of 4% compared with the best previous reported performance using conventional methods of 88% and 26%, respectively.

In cytology ANNs have been compared with conventional techniques with the aim of automating the identification of pre-cancerous cervical cells.[41] A frequency domain approach was used to compute a discriminant function that was used to classify the cells as normal or abnormal. This was compared with a conventional morphology approach that used various parameters, including the area of nucleus/area of cytoplasm ratio. Both methods were compared with the back-propagation network using 80 features derived from the frequency domain. Of the three methods the morphology approach was the best with 99% accuracy and 3.8% maximum false-negative results, while using identical data the frequency domain approach gave 98% accuracy and the ANN 95%. Thus ANNs are not necessarily the best method to use, and conventional techniques should be considered, and where appropriate used as a comparison for ANNs. However, if accuracy may be compromised, the ANN may be less labour intensive than a conventional approach.

A priori knowledge

Networks tend to work rather badly without some external help. This is hardly surprising. The brain is a complicated set of systems that work co-operatively. To solve a problem you might use several senses. Giving the ANN as much information as possible, rather than simply placing raw data in its input layer, usually improves performance.

Rather than parameterizing ECG readings, Lee[42] used digitized patterns. There is a problem inherent in this approach, i.e. it will not be known a priori where the QRS starts. One could pre-process the data to determine where the QRS is located, but the network was made to be translation independent. A trained MLN was able to distinguish with high accuracy between normal sinus rhythm, ventricular tachycardia and ventricular fibrillation.

Evoked EEG potentials have been used to classify neurological diseases.[43] It was suggested that the ANN needed to be supplemented with additional knowledge to diagnose accurately, and that this could be implemented by pre-processing the data or by building a cooperative system. The former approach would recognize 'well-behaved' patterns and process them in an ANN. The latter approach would take the results from an ANN and combine them with other data to effect a diagnosis.

Generalizability

The network may give a good solution for a training set of data, but not have learned the general solution. In other words, it may have learned the specific training case, but not similar ones. To test whether the network has generalized you need to present a test set of data which the network was not trained on. If the network gives a similar performance on these data as on training data you can be reasonably sure that the network has really 'learned' the solution. If the training data set is accurately classified, but not the test set, the ANN has learned the wrong solution.

An analogy should make this clearer. A small child is told that Rover, the labrador, is a dog. The next time she is shown Rover she says 'dog', but when shown Butch, the terrier, she does not know what to call him. She has not generalized the concept of dog, but knows the particular case of Rover. When she realizes that not just Rover, but all labradors, are 'dog' she still has the wrong answer; it is only when all dogs are correctly classified that she has got the concept. One important thing to note is that the child cannot be expected to remember each dog, rather she develops a concept whereby a totally new breed she has never seen before would probably be classified correctly as a dog.

It is possible for ANNs to learn that a particular set of numbers from an image mean that the cells in the image are cancerous and that another set of numbers mean that the cells are not cancerous. However, when shown new image data the network gets it all wrong. This can happen with *one-to-one mapping*, where the specific numbers are learned, rather than the general concept.

The solution is to have more data than the ANN can store, so that it has 'no choice' but to generalize. An empirical observation is that one should have fewer connections than patterns, and this should not only dissuade one-to-one mappings, but also greatly speed up the training.[44] However, Hart[45] states, this may not be sufficient. For the test set to be of any use certain criteria should be met:

- *Repeatability*. The data collected should have low within observer and between observer error
- *Representativity*. An adequate amount of data for each class should be present
- *Accuracy*. The data should be as complete as possible, and each item should be as accurate as possible.

As the test data may not be sufficient to allow generalization (e.g. the data may be difficult or expensive to generate), one solution is to add 'noise' (random error) onto each data pattern so that the ANN does not get exactly the same inputs each time it is trained on a pattern.

The black box

One of the limitations of ANNs is the difficulty in determining what is happening within the network. The ANN is typically treated as a 'black box', with known inputs and outputs that are, hopefully, appropriate to the problem under study. Using a 'black box', where this is defined to be a system the inputs and outputs of which are examinable, but the internal workings of which are obscure, is appropriate where the relationships between inputs and outputs are not well known, provided one is aware of certain problems.

While the internal functioning of the network is difficult to analyse, some work has been done to gain some idea of what is going on. Rules may be generated from an expert system network. This may be achieved[16,46] by setting all inputs 'off', and monitoring the effect of the output states of diseases on the trained network. Where an additional input is turned on that switches the output off again, a negative rule is obtained. Combinatorial explosion may be avoided by limiting the number of affirmative and negative components to a rule. A list of rules drawn up in this fashion was judged by medically trained personnel to be reasonable.

If the classification of patterns is taken as the sole criterion of success of an ANN, one may get an undesirable performance for specific problems. For example, it is more important to avoid misdiagnosing serious head injury as a psychosomatic illness, than vice versa, and therefore a network may need to show a worse absolute classification rate to avoid disastrous misdiagnoses. The prognosis of head injury has been explored using an ANN system.[47] A cost matrix was used to penalize the misclassifications that it is most important to get right.

In a medical system, where the outputs may be used to make decisions that could be critical to a patient, the effects of errors are pertinent. In an expert system, for example, one may analyse the effects of incorrect data entry by flipping the state of the input from a correct to an incorrect value, and determining the effect of this change on the resultant output, which may be, say, a diagnosis.[48]

In many cases there is no true gold standard to compare an ANN with, other than the opinion of clinicians, but they could of course be wrong. In these cases, where there are some discrepancies between the rules generated by doctors and those generated by the MLP, it may be worth reconsidering the medical judgements, rather than assuming that the MLP is wrong. Thus the MLP may be seen as a useful indicator of possible clinical rule adjustments.

In most of the studies described above, ANNs were trained in 'supervised' mode. This means that training data sets with target outputs were given to the ANN. In many cases it is difficult and expensive to obtain sufficiently large data sets. Furthermore, the targets are often assigned by subjective assessment (e.g. a physician's diagnosis) and may not be correct. Unsupervised learning may be achieved via ANNs. Kohonen nets[49] take input data and arrange them into classes, with no supervision. More conventional unsupervised classification techniques include the k-means method.

Overtraining

If an ANN is trained beyond the point of convergence, the total error may still be falling slightly, but the classification of unseen data may become worse.[50] The training data are subject to overfitting after convergence, and generally this should be avoided. One technique for spotting this is to use a test set to report an error, but not to use it in training. In other words, a training set that is different from the test set is used to update the weights. Overfitting will be evident from an increased test set error.

Large problems

ANNs scale badly; the time taken to converge is empirically related to the cube of the number of links.[44] So splitting a problem up into smaller problems to be solved by subnetworks is highly desirable. Another method is to reduce the number of inputs by data compression. A separate neural network can actually be used to perform the compression. A set of inputs is fed into a much smaller number of units in the second 'hidden' layer; the data are fed out into the output layer, which has the same number of units as the input layer. The network is trained to give an output that is identical to the input. Once trained the output layer can be removed, and the hidden layer contains a reduced dimension representation of the input layer.

For example, data compression using an MLP has been used to reduce the data of a digital Holter monitor. The network construction was similar to earlier work[51] where an MLP learned the identity mapping, using inputs as targets, and a single hidden layer gave a reduced dimensional representation of the data. Nagasaka et al[52] have monitored the error of the trained network in real time, while training a second network on current data. If the error of reconstructing the data frequently went above a given threshold, the second network was copied to the original network, and thereafter used as the compressor. All networks were saved along with the outputs of the hidden layer, which may later be used to reconstruct the data.

Which ANN to use

For any given problem there are frequently several choices of ANN available. For example, arterial pressure waveforms have been analysed using two different ANN paradigms: back-propagation and competitive learning.[53] In the latter there is unsupervised learning, i.e. there is no 'teacher' involved. The back-propagation net successfully classified all test patterns as artefact or artefact-free. The competitive model had a high success rate of 93%, but consistently missed artefacts, classifying them as artefact-free. However, it is difficult to see how this could have been known a priori.

Design of the network

Generally networks are designed by trial and error, as they are notoriously difficult to design analytically. For example, you need to know how many hidden layers you should have, the necessary number of units in each layer, and what connections should there be among the units and layers. Empirically it is thought that having more than one hidden layer is not useful. Some work has been done using genetic algorithms to find optimal structures.[54] Networks may also be pruned of nodes where the least utility is located.[55]

Initial parameters

Networks can learn quickly and possibly badly, or slowly and (hopefully) more accurately (see the section on simulated annealing earlier in this chapter). The speed is defined by the 'learning rate', which needs to be set low for large networks. A high learning rate in large networks causes 'flooding' of the hidden layers, whereby they become fixed at constant and incorrect values. Slower learning rates are less likely to cause flooding, but of course it takes longer to arrive at a solution. Unfortunately, the learning rate is just one of the parameters used in back-propagation ANNs (parameters of various sorts are used in most other designs also). Momentum is another, whereby the changes in weights are smoothed out by always including a part of the previous weight change.

ANNs are sensitive to the initial conditions and the parameters used (e.g. momentum and learning rate). The parameters used are often arrived at by trial and error, although some work has been done on automatically setting the parameters and tuning them dynamically to the current state of the network.[56-58]

Noisy input

It is generally stated that ANNs are resistant to 'noise' and erroneous inputs, although rarely is this aspect covered in actual implementations. It has been shown that ANNs trained on noiseless data are not as resistant to noise as those trained on data with noise. Thus in simulations, exact derived data may not be adequate for training a system that will use real data. If the network itself, as opposed to the data input to it, is likely to be subject to corruption, the network may need to be overtrained. In simulations, nets that had been trained past convergence were more hardware resistant than were those for which training had stopped at convergence.[59]

The information becomes more evenly spread through the network after convergence is reached. Thus one may wish to effect a compromise between fault tolerance and overtraining if faults in hardware are likely.

GENETIC ALGORITHMS

Genetic algorithms (GAs) are based on the theory of genetics, and are not neural networks, but have a similar usage, and therefore will be briefly discussed in this chapter. An overview of GAs is given in De Jong.[60] The basic idea is that the solution to a problem evolves over time. The concepts of evolution are used in a simulation. There are simulated genes, which are binary strings (zeros and ones), and these strings can 'mutate' by randomly switching a zero to a one, or vice versa. Two strings can exchange portions and produce 'offspring' (probably the cleanest 'simulated sex' ever seen).

The synthetic genes are tested in some manner for 'fitness' and those that perform best are permitted more offspring. It is beyond the scope of this text to describe the details of specifying fitness, etc., and you are referred to texts such as those by De Jong[60] and Grenfenstette.[61] There are computer packages available, often for no cost, e.g. GENESIS (not to be confused with the neural network package of the same name).[62]

Examples of the use of GAs includes teaching a pair of sticks to 'walk'.[63] However, of particular relevance to this chapter is that GAs have been used to design neural networks. The philosophy behind this might be that genetics designed the real neural networks (e.g. the brains of humans). Neural network architecture is notoriously difficult to optimize using analytic techniques, and neural networks are usually designed using empirical methods (i.e. 'suck it and see'). It is not illogical, therefore, to use artificial genetics to build artificial neural networks. This has been achieved with some success[64,65] on small 'toy' problems, although when I tried it on a larger problem it did not perform well.[66] However, the problems were quite different in type as well as size, and it remains to be seen whether this technique can be used generally to design networks.

EXAMPLE: A NEURAL NETWORK APPLICATION – PRESSURE SORE PREDICTION

A logistic regression model (see Ch. 7) was built using the forward conditional method in SPSS, with all 11 variables of the Waterlow scale used initially. Only three variables were kept in the logistic regression formula: appetite, continence and skin. MLPs were computed for all 11 variables as inputs, with both 11 and five hidden units. Purely linear networks were also created using no hidden units. All simulations were completed using NevProp version 3.0.[1]

Using the training data, ROC curves (see Ch. 8) showed that the best fit was for

Table 11.1   Training data

Test	Area under ROC curve (c index)
MLP 11 inputs, 11 hidden units	0.9984
MLP 11 inputs, 5 hidden units	0.9945
Linear net 11 inputs	0.9472
Logistic regression	0.9276
Linear net 3 inputs	0.8273

the most complex network, an MLP with all variables used as inputs and with 11 hidden units (Table 11.1). However, a problem with ANNs is that a solution that works well on training data will not necessarily be generalizable. In the worst possible case a one-to-one mapping is created where the network stores the information necessary to recreate the data set, but not the general concepts. This is most likely to occur with larger networks and smaller training sets.

The solution is to have more data than the ANN can store, so that it has 'no choice' but to generalize. An empirical observation is that one should have fewer connections than patterns, and this should not only prevent one-to-one mappings, but greatly speeds up the training.[44] With 11 inputs, 11 hidden units and one output unit the number of connections is 132. The number of patterns in the training set was 211, which should be sufficient to allow generalization. The other networks were smaller still.

By adding arbitrarily complex transformations one may always fit some formula to any data. If the transformations are not representative of real characteristics of the data set, this simply results in overfitting of the data. In this case the overfitted model may not only be more complex, but may perform less well on new data. However well the network performs on training data, the real test is how well it classifies unseen test data. A particular problem with ANNs is that, as training of the network proceeds, beyond a certain point the network is no longer learning, but overfitting, and the network is said to be overtrained.

If an ANN is trained beyond the point of convergence, the total error may still be falling slightly, but the classification of unseen data may become worse.[50] The training data are subject to overfitting after convergence, and generally this should be avoided. One technique to spot this is to use a test set to report an error, but not to use it in training; i.e. a training set is used to update the weights that is separate from the test set. Overfitting will be evident from an increased test set error. NevProp uses the test set to ascertain how many iterations to use on the training set.

Using test data the rank order of the tests is virtually reversed. It now appears that the most complex ANNs using non-linearities score least well, and while the MLP with 11 hidden units performed better than the one with five, the difference is small. Reducing the number of inputs, i.e. using a subset of the input data (the three variables of continence, appetite and skin), actually performs better on test

Table 11.2   Test data

Test	Area under ROC curve (c index)
Logistic regression 3 variables	0.854666
Linear regression 3 variables	0.849832
Linear net 11 inputs	0.817465
Linear net 3 inputs	0.813892
MLP 3 hidden units, 3 inputs	0.806536
MLP 11 inputs, 11 hidden units	0.7899
MLP 11 inputs, 5 hidden units	0.76219

data. A purely linear network with all 11 inputs and no hidden units, and one with only the three inputs perform similarly and better than any of the non-linear MLPs. Finally, linear regression and logistic regression done with the three variables found in a logistic regression analysis to be significant, perform best of all (Table 11.2).

In this study only three of the variables showed a significant predictive ability: continence, skin assessment and appetite. Using the other variables in a linear network improved the predictive ability of the network only marginally. A logistic regression performed better than any network, and in particular non-linear networks did not offer a better solution. It would appear, based on this moderately sized sample, that in elderly inpatients a linear combination of the variables of the Waterlow score are as effective, if not more so, than a more complex non-linear solution.

The linear solution offered by a linear regression analysis was:

$$\text{Sore} = (\text{APPETITE} \times 0.054) + (\text{CONTINENCE} \times 0.064) + (\text{SKIN} \times 0.14) - 0.066$$

The linear network also gave weights connecting the inputs to the (single) output which were similar for appetite and continence and roughly double for skin. This is unsurprising as the network is trying to fit a linear solution to the problem. The NevProp network simulator also reports the relevance of each of the inputs as a percentage, and it gave skin assessment roughly two-thirds (67%) of the relevance, and less than 10% to the other two items, even when all 11 inputs were used. Thus it would seem that the assessment of skin is the main item of the Waterlow score that gives it a predictive ability. This indicates that the values for skin assessment are roughly twice as important as those for appetite or continence. If this is generally the case, the Waterlow score should have a wider range of value for skin assessment (say by doubling the score).

This study should not be seen to show that ANNs are not appropriate in this form of analysis, but rather that in this case a non-linear solution did not out-perform a linear one. The problem under study can be modelled as a linear problem, and thus a more complex non-linear solution is neither required nor able to improve on the prediction offered by the simpler technique.

CONCLUSION

ANNs are a useful technique for solving problems that traditional sequential computer programs are not good at, but that humans (and other animals) often perform with apparent ease. They do not necessarily outperform simpler linear methods, and should only be used if they show a demonstrable improvement in performance. Inherently non-linear problems are typical candidates for neural network solutions.

REFERENCES

1. Goodman P H 1996 NevProp software, version 3. University of Nevada, Reno NV
2. Lawler 1976 Combinatorial optimization: Networks and matroids. Holt Rinehart and Winston, New York
3. Garey M R, Johnson D S 1979 Computers and intractability. W H Freeman, San Francisco, CA
4. Hebb D O 1949 The organization of behavior. Wiley, New York
5. Aarts E, Korst J 1989 Simulated annealing and Boltzmann machines. Wiley, New York
6. Kirkpatrick S, Gelatt C D 1983 Optimisation by simulated annealing. Science 220: 671–680
7. Rumelhart D E, Hinton G E, Williams N 1986 Learning internal representations by error propagation. In (Rumelhart D E, McLelland J L eds) Parallel distributed processing. MIT Press, Cambridge, MA, p 318–362
8. Kolonay M A, Klimasauskas C C 1987 An introduction to neural computing. NeuralWare Professional,
9. Chan L 1989 Adaptive and invariant connectionist models for pattern recognition. PhD thesis, Cambridge University Engineering Department, UK
10. Rosenblatt F 1959 Two theorems of statistical separability in the perceptron. In: Mechanisation of thought processes: Proceedings of a symposium held at the National Physical Laboratory. HMSO, London, p 421–456
11. Minsky M L, Papert S 1969 Perceptrons. MIT Press, Cambridge, MA
12. Minsky M L, Papert S 1988 Perceptrons, expanded edn. MIT Press, Cambridge, MA
13. Rumelhart D E, McLelland J L 1986 Parallel distributed processing. MIT Press, Cambridge, MA
14. Anthony D M 1994 Appropriate use of neural networks in medical imaging. In: Neural net and expert systems in medicine and healthcare. University of Plymouth, UK, p 45–52
15. Hart A, Yyatt J 1989 Connectionist models in medicine: An investigation of their potential. In: Hunter J, Yyatt J (eds) Lecture notes in medical informatics. Springer-Verlag, Berlin, p 115–124
16. Saito K, Nakano R 1988 Medical diagnostic expert system based on PDP model. In: IEEE Proceeding of the International Conference on neural networks, San Diego, CA, Vol 1, p 255–262
17. Baxt W G 1990 Use of artificial neural network for data analysis in clinical decision-making: The diagnosis of acute coronary occlusion. Neural Computation 2: 480–489
18. Cohen M E, Hudson D L, Anderson M F 1989 Combination of a neural model and a rule-based expert system to determine efficacy of medical testing procedures. In: Images of the 21st Century: IEEE Engineering in Medicine and Biology 11th Annual Conference, IEEE, Seattle
19. Neaves P 1991 Design and development of a complex impedance measurement system for impedance tomography. MSc thesis, Warwick University, UK
20. Egbert D D, Rhodes E E 1988 Preprocessing of biomedical images for neurocomputer analysis. In: IEEE Proceedings of the Conference on Neural Network, IEEE, San Diego, CA, p 561–568
21. Cheung J Y, Hull Jr S S 1989 Detection of abnormal electrocardiograms using a neural

network approach. In: Images of the 21st century: IEEE Engineering in Medicine and Biology 11th Annual Conference, IEEE, Seattle, p 2015–2016

22. Pietka E 1989 Neural nets for ECG classification. In: Images of the 21st century: IEEE Engineering in Medicine and Biology 11th Annual Conference, IEEE, Seattle, p 2021–2022

23. Xue Q, Hu Y, Tompkins W J 1989 A neural network weight pattern study with ECG pattern recognition. In: Images of the 21st Century: IEEE Engineering in Medicine and Biology 11th Annual Conference, IEEE, Seattle, p 2023–2024

24. Eberhart R C, Dobbins R W, Webber W R S 1989 EEG waveform analysis using casenet. In: Images of the 21st Century: IEEE Engineering in Medicine and Biology 11th Annual Conference, IEEE, Seattle, p 2046–2057

25. Hiraiwa A, Shimohara K, Tokunaga Y 1989 EEG topography recognition by neural network IEEE International Conference on Systems, Man, and Cybernetics, vol 3, IEEE, Cambridge, MA p 1116–1117

26. Sochor H, Dorffner G, Porenta G 1988 Classification of thallium-201 scintigrams using a neural network trained by back propagation. Journal of Nuclear Medicine 29(7): 1314

27. Anthony D M 1991 The use of artificial neural networks in classifying lung scintigrams. PhD Dissertation, University of Warwick, UK

28. Ozkan H, Hendrick M S, Sprenkels G, Benoit M S, Dawant M 1990 Multi-spectral magnetic resonance image segmentation using neural networks. In: 4th IJCNN International Joint Conference on Neural Networks. IEEE, San Diego, CA, vol 1, p 429–434

29. Grossberg S, Mingolla E 1985 Neural dynamics of perceptual grouping: Textures boundaries and emergent segmentation. Perception and Psychophysics 38: 144–210

30. Lehar S M, Worth A J, Kennedy D N 1990 Application of the boundary contour/feature contour system to magnetic resonance brain scan imagery. In: 4th IJCNN International Joint Conference on Neural Networks, IEEE, San Diego, CA, vol 1, p 435–440

31. Boone J M, Sigillito V G, Shaber G S 1990 Neural networks in radiology: An introduction and evaluation in a signal detection task. Medical Physics 17(2): 234–241

32. Baker B, Curry S, Baumrind S 1989 Neural network method for solving pattern recognition problems in craniofacial X-ray image analysis. In: Image of the 21st Century: IEEE Engineering in Medicine and Biology 11th Annual Conference, vol 11(5), IEEE, Seattle p 1646

33. Shadmehr R, D'Argenio D Z 1989 Connectionist Modeling vs Bayesian procedures for sparse data pharmokinetic parameter estimation. In: Images of the 21st Century: IEEE Engineering in Medicine and Biology 11th Annual Conference, IEEE, Seattle p 2058–2059

34. Shadmehr R 1990 A neural network for nonlinear Bayesian estimation in drug therapy. Neural Computation 2: 216–225

35. Microcompter Centre 1990 Research bulletin. Microcomputer Centre, University of Dundee, UK

36. Anthony D M, Hines E L, Taylor D, Barham J 1989 An investigation into the use of neural networks for an expert system in nuclear medicine image analysis. In: IEE 3rd International Conference on Image Processing and its Applications, Warwick University, IEE, Coventry, UK, p 338–342

37. Anthony D M, Hines E L, Hutchins D, Mottram T 1991 Simulated tomography ultrasound imaging of defects. In: Taylor J G (ed) Neural networks applications. Springer-Verlag, London

38. Conrath B C, Daft C M W, O'Brien W D 1989 Applications of neural networks to ultrasound tomography. In: IEEE Ultrasonics Symposium, IEEE, Montreal p 1007–1010

39. Watanabe S, Yoneyama M 1990 Ultrasonic robot eyes using neural networks. IEEE Transactions on Ultrasonics, Ferroelectrics and Frequency Control 37: 141–147

40. Nikoonahad M, Liu D C 1990 Medical ultrasound imaging using neural networks. Electronic Letters 26(8): 545–546

41. Ricketts I W 1990 Neural networks and conventional approaches to the detection of abnormal cells. Department of Mathematics and Computer Science, University of Dundee, UK

42. Lee S C 1989 A neural network weight pattern study with ECG pattern recognition. In:

Images of the 21st Century: IEEE Engineering in Medicine and Biology 11th Annual
Conference, IEEE, Seattle, p 2025–2026

43. Bruha I, Madhaven G P 1989 Need for a knowledge-based subsystem in evoked
potential neural-net recognition system. In: Images of the 21st Century: IEEE
Engineering in Medicine and Biology 11th Annual Conference, IEEE, Seattle p 2042–2043

44. Hinton G E 1989 Connectionist learning procedures. Artificial Intelligence 40: 185–234

45. Hart A 1990 Evaluating black boxes as medical decision aids. Medical Informatics 15(3):
229–236

46. Saito K, Nakano R 1990 Rule extraction from facts and neural networks. In: INNS
International Neural Networks Conference, INNS, Paris, vol 1, p 379–382

47. Lowe D, Webb A 1990 Exploiting prior knowledge in network optimization: An
illustration from medical prognosis. Network 1: 199–323

48. Hyman W A, Mitta D A 1989 Statistical analysis of the effect of input errors on expert
system advice. In: Images of the 21st Century: IEEE Engineering in Medicine and
Biology 11th Annual Conference, IEEE, Seattle, p 1771–1772

49. Kohonen T 1982 Self organized formation of topologically correct feature maps.
Biological Cybernetics 43: 59–69

50. Chauvin Y 1987 Generalization performance of overtrained back-propagation networks.
In: Almeida L B, Wellekens C J (eds) Neural networks. Springer-Verlag, Berlin, p 46–55

51. Cottrell G W, Munro P, Zipser D 1987 Learning internal representations from gray-scale
images: An example of extensional programming. In: Cognitive Science Society Annual
Conference, 9th Proceedings, Seattle, W A, p 461–473

52. Nagasaka Y, Iwata A, Suzumura N 1989 Data compression using neural network for
digital holter monitor. In: Images of the 21st Centruy: IEEE Engineering in Medicine and
Biology 11th Annual Conference, IEEE, Seattle, p 2019–2020

53. Sebald A V, Mitta D A 1989 Use of neural networks for detection of artifacts in arterial
pressure waveforms. In: Images of the 21st Century: IEEE Engineering in Medicine and
Biology 11th Annual Conference, IEEE, Seattle, p 2034–2035

54. Harp, S A, Samad T, Guha A 1989 Towards the genetic synthesis of neural networks. In:
3rd International Conference on Genetic Algorithms, George Mason University Fairfax,
VA, MIT, Cambridge, MA, p 360–369

55. Sankar A, Mammone R J 1990 Optimal pruning of neural tree networks for improved
generalization. In: IJCNN International Joint Conference on Neural Networks, IJCNN,
Seattle, WA, Vol 1, p219–224

56. Lister J B, Schnurrenberger H, Mamillod P 1990 Implementation of a multi-layer
perceptron for a non-linear control problem. Ecole Polytechnique Federale de Lausanne

57. Vogl T P, Mangis J K, Rigler A K, Zink W T, Alkon D L 1988 Accelerating the
convergence of the back-propagation method. Biological Cybernetics 59: 257–263

58. Chan L, Fallside F 1987 An adaptive training algorithm for back propagation networks.
Computer Speech and Language 2: 205–218

59. Nijhuis J, Spaanenburg L 1989 Fault tolerance of neural associative memories. IEE
Proceedings 136(E): 389–394

60. De Jong K 1980 Adaptive system design: A genetic approach. IEEE Transactions on
Ultrasonics, Ferroelectrics and Frequency Control SMC-10(9): 566–574

61. Holland J 1987 Genetic algorithms and classifier systems: foundations and future
directions. In: proceedings of the International Conference on Genetic Algorithms, MIT,
Cambridge, MA, p 82–89

62. Grenfenstette J J 1984 A user's guide to GENESIS. Computer Science Department
Vanderbilt University, Nashville, TN, technical report CS-84–11

63. De Garis H 1989 WALKER, a genetically programmed, time dependent, neural net
which teaches a pair of sticks to walk. Center for AI, George Mason University Virginia
VA, technical report

64. Schaffer J D, Caruana R A, Eshelman L J 1989 Using genetic search to exploit the
emergent behavior of neural networks. Phillips Labs, New York, technical report p 1–8

65. Miller G F, Todd P M, Hegde S U 1989 Designing neural networks using genetic
algorithms. In: 3rd International Conference on Genetic Algorithms, George Mason
University, Fairfax, VA. MIT, Cambridge, MA, p 379–384

66. Anthony D M 1991 The use of artificial neural networks in classifying lung scintigrams.
Ph D Dissertation, University of Warwick, UK, p 121–130

12

Power analysis: how large should a sample be?

Introduction	Power of a test
Surveys	**Exercises**
Power analysis Type I error Type II error Effect	**Conclusion** **References**

When you are planning a study you need to know how many subjects to recruit. If your sample is too small you risk missing a real effect (Type II error), but if your sample is larger than needed it presents economic (it is expensive to perform large studies) and ethical (why perform experiments on people for no good reason) problems. This chapter looks at methods of selecting the optimal sample size for your work.

KEY POINTS

- Samples are estimates of populations
- The sample size required for a given accuracy is independent of the population size
- Statistics tests vary in their power, i.e. their ability to detect a real effect
- Statistical and clinical signicance are not the same thing

At the end of this chapter the student should be able to:

1. *Estimate the sample size required given certain information about the population*
2. *Understand the difference between statistical and clinical signicance*
3. *Given certain parameters, estimate the effect observable for a given sample size, or the sample size needed to observe a given effect*

INTRODUCTION

One of the questions most commonly asked by students undertaking a research project is 'How many subjects do I need?' Most texts give general guidelines on the size of a sample, which is in essence:

- the bigger the sample the better
- there is an increased cost and a diminishing return as the number of subjects gets larger.

However, under most circumstances it is possible to give a more precise estimate of the sample size needed to test a hypothesis. For an excellent text on this subject for inferential tests see Cohen,[1] and for sample sizes in descriptive surveys see Stuart.[2]

SURVEYS

If you are doing a survey using purely descriptive statistics, i.e. you are not performing any inferential tests, then you still need at least a sample size that is representative of the population at large, or your description will not inform you about the larger population.

A classic sampling problem is to estimate the sample size needed to predict an election. In this case we are interested in the percentage of a sample that would vote for a particular party, and we require it to be accurate to within, say, 5%. Alternatively, we may have a sample, or series of samples, and want to know to what level of confidence we may attribute the results.

Another typical requirement is to have a sample that will probably be within so many percent of the true population with respect to some parameter (e.g. the mean value). If we are attempting to measure some (typically interval/ratio) variable in the population, we will only have the estimate from our sample. If another sample is taken it will give an estimate that will almost certainly be slightly different from that from the first sample. Thus, in addition to the variance of the individual values, the *population variance*, the sample varies also. The variance in the samples is naturally named the *sample variance* and is a measure of the fluctuations in the mean values of different samples. The *standard error of the mean* (SEM) is simply the square root of the sample variance. Thus the SEM is analogous to the *standard deviation*; while the latter measures variability among individuals in the population, the former measures variability among samples.

The variance of the sample reduces as the sample becomes larger, and when the sample is the population, i.e. we sample the whole population, the variance will clearly be zero, as no variation is possible in such a case. You might consider that the sampling variance is strongly connected to the population size. Fortunately, in large populations this is *not* true, and is in fact related to the sample size, almost regardless of the population size. The variance of the sample is approximately[3] that of the population variance multiplied by $(N - n)/[n(N - 1)]$, where N is the population size and n is the sample size. When N is much bigger than n this ratio becomes close to $1/n$, which leads us to the interesting conclusion that the sampling variance is not dependent on the population size at all, provided the population is much larger than the sample size. If the adult population of the UK (ca. 40 million) is our population and a sample of 200 is measured for, say, blood pressure, then the more complicated exact formula will give almost exactly the same results as the simpler formula.

Often we wish to estimate some parameter (typically an interval/ratio value such as height or weight) in a population where we are unable to measure the whole population but have access to a small sample of the population. Suppose we wanted to determine the average height of our students. We might expect them to be higher than the national average, as the majority are middle class, and in general the middle class are taller than the working class, with the latter probably being a proxy for poverty. In fact there are significant differences in all European countries for height against class, except for the Republic of Ireland. Suppose we wanted to determine a mean height to within 1 inch (about 2.5 cm). Suppose further that the standard deviation of height in the university was known to be 5 cm (this is fictional data). Finally, we want to be 95% sure of our results. What sample size would we need?

We want to know how many of our students to measure to get a reasonable value for height. The standard error of the mean (SEM) measures the variance of the mean values taken from a population. We know that 95% of the sample means in a normal distribution fall within about 2 SEM. Thus if two standard errors are to equal 2.5 cm, which is our criterion, the standard error should be about 2.5/2, or 1.25 units. The sampling variance, which is the square of the standard error, is thus about 1.56. Since the sampling variance is given above as population variance divided by the number in the sample, to ascertain the sample size n, we need

$$\text{Sampling variance} = \frac{\text{Population variance}}{n}$$

Rearranging the above gives

$$n = \frac{\text{Population variance}}{\text{Sampling variance}}$$

The population variance is the square of the standard deviation or about 25, so

$$n = \frac{25}{1.56} = 16.0$$

(to one decimal place). Thus we would need about sixteen subjects to be within about 2.5 cm (in fact if we used exact arithmetic, using 1.5625 for the sample variance rather than rounding it down to 1.56, the result is exactly 16). Increasing the precision to half an inch, or about 1.25 cm, we would need a sample size with a standard error of 0.625 units, which will give

$$n = \frac{25}{0.625^2} = 64$$

So doubling the precision from 2.5 to 1.25 cm involves quadrupling the number of subjects from 16 to 64. This is a general rule, and increasing the sample size does therefore not result in a corresponding linear increase in precision. There is a law of diminishing returns: precision is related to the square of the sample size (the relationship is, not linear), so sample size quickly becomes prohibitive for unnecessarily high precision. To keep the sample size small (and cheap) you need to have a realistic idea of the precision you actually need, rather than what you might want in an ideal world.

In many cases precision can be improved with no extra sampling by careful selection of the sample, in particular by dividing samples into strata or clusters. For further details you should refer to a specialist book on this topic, such as the one by Stuart.[2]

POWER ANALYSIS

Type I error

This form of error occurs when the statistical test gives a probability below that of the alpha value (α), thus indicating that the null hypothesis is false when it is in fact true. This does not necessarily mean that any mistake has been made by the investigator. It is the nature of statistics that it deals in the probability of a result being significant. If there is a p value of 0.05, it means that you could have got this result by chance only 1 time in 20 (5%). When in fact you do get such a result by chance, rather than because of a genuine effect (a true difference between the means in a Student's t-test, a real correlation, etc.) this is a type I error. A type I error can be minimized by reducing the α value, and the probability of getting a type I error is precisely the α value that you elect to have. Thus if you choose to have an α value of 0.01 ($\alpha = 0.01$) then you will get fewer (a fifth as many) type I errors than with $\alpha = 0.05$. So reducing the α value by definition reduces type I errors.

Type II error

Unfortunately it is also possible to get the opposite problem, where the null hypothesis is false but your test fails to reject it. If you set a very low α value you are more likely to find no effect, even if it exists, especially if your sample size is small. If a test gives a p value of 0.02, say, then with $\alpha = 0.05$ the null hypothesis is rejected, but with $\alpha = 0.01$ it is accepted. Thus, with $\alpha = 0.01$, even though there is only a 2% chance that the results came about purely by chance, the apparent effect (the difference between the means of two groups, say) is assumed not to be significant. If the sample size is small, getting below such a small probability as 0.01 might be difficult or even impossible. With small samples the differences in means (or size of correlations, etc.) need to be large to be significant; conversely, a low α value with small sample sizes will not detect small effects even if they are real. Thus to avoid type II errors you should raise the α level.

Effect

The difference between the mean values for two groups or the size of a correlation coefficient, for example, are of at least as much interest as the statistical significance of the test result. If a highly significant result ($p < 0.01$, say) indicates a real but tiny difference in the healing rates of wounds under different dressings, or minute differences in the serum glucose levels for two diabetic regimes, then clinical significance may be minor or absent. Typically such a scenario occurs with very large samples. Conversely, a very large difference between groups, say, which may be highly significant clinically may be of a lesser statistical significance, and possibly not significant at all if the sample size is very small. So statistical significance tells us how confident we are of a result, not how important the results are, while clinical significance tells us how much (or even whether) we care about the result, but says nothing about the confidence we have in our results.

The clinical significance is measured by an *effect*. Quite what constitutes an effect varies depending on the test under discussion. Some examples are:

- *Differences between groups*. The effect will be the difference between the mean values if the data are normally distributed. However, since the raw data will be sensitive to the measuring scale (a difference of 1 m is clearly not the same as a difference of 1 foot), we standardize the effect by using z scores (differences measured in standard deviations), which are not sensitive to the actual scales used and will give identical results whether measured in metres or inches, or in kilograms or grains.

- *Differences in frequencies*. Nominal data cannot be given a mean value, but often we want to assess the divergence of observed frequencies against what we would have expected by chance. Such a measure is w, which is discussed below.

- *Correlations*. The value of the correlation coefficient r is used as an effect measure. A low value ($r = 0.1$) means that 1% of the variance of one variable is apparently explained by the other, but a high value ($r = 0.5$) means that 25% of the variance of one variable is apparently explained by the other. (There is also an effect for looking at the differences between correlations; however, first the difference needs transforming into a z score, which is achieved by using a table of transformations from r to z; see Cohen.[4])
- *Sign test*. The difference between a $0.50 : 0.50$ split in the ratios of positives and negatives (which would be an effect of zero) and any other split indicates the strength of the effect. So a $0.90 : 0.10$ split would be an effect of 0.4 (as it is 0.4 away from the null result).

Power of a test

Different tests have varying ability to give a positive result. In other words when the null hypothesis is false, one test may (correctly) reject it while a similar test will fail to reject the null hypothesis. Thus at a given α value one test fails to discriminate between a real effect, while the other detects it. The latter test is said to have greater power. Since investigators clearly want to use a test that tells them that an effect is real when in fact it is, they will want a more powerful test when there is a choice of more than one test. In general, parametric tests are more powerful than non-parametric tests, and this leads some researchers to use the parametric test in all cases. This is not sensible if the conditions of the test are violated (typically using the test on severely skewed non-normal distributions) when the results of the test may be meaningless. Thus you should use the most powerful test that is allowed given your data type and distribution.

If the probability of accepting the null hypothesis when it is false (i.e. the probability of a type II error) is β, then clearly the probability of correctly rejecting the null hypothesis must be $1 - \beta$. We want $1 - \beta$, which we call the power of the test, to be as high as possible for a given test, and its maximum value will be unity.

Power curves can be computed, which show the relationship of $1 - \beta$ with the effect.[5] If we were looking at the difference between mean values then the effect would be $(\mu_1 - \mu_2)/\sigma$, where μ_1 is the mean of one group, μ_2 is the mean of the other group and σ is the standard deviation (assumed here to be calculated from the data for both groups combined). For each possible effect $(\mu_1 - \mu_2)/\sigma$ there will be a different value of $1 - \beta$. When in fact the two means are the same ($\mu_1 = \mu_2$) there is still a possibility that the test will report them as different, i.e. our samples gave estimates of μ_1 and μ_2 that are different from the real μ_1 and μ_2 due to random (chance) variations that were incorrectly evaluated by the test as significant.

Cohen[1] gives *power tables* for a variety of tests. These tables give the effect sizes detectable for a given test and sample size and various α values. Thus if you knew the effect size that you were looking for, you can determine the sample size needed to detect such an effect for a given α value at a given power. The power you choose will have a major impact on the sample size. Cohen[6] advocates a power of 0.8 as a suitable power value to use by default. The rationale for this is that a power close to unity is virtually impossible to achieve, and very expensive if it is possible at all. A power of 0.8 means, by definition, that $\beta = 0.2$. Thus we are implicitly saying that we consider a type II error (failing to detect an effect when it exists) is about one-fourth as serious as a type 1 error (falsely stating an effect to exist when no effect exists). As α is typically set to 0.05, which is four times more stringent than $\beta = 0.2$, this seems a priori reasonable, in that we need to be more sure when stating that an effect exists than when rejecting an effect as due to random error. While you may think the two values should logically be the same, in practice positive results are more likely to get published than negative ones, so some prejudice against type I error may be considered acceptable.

In practice you will not always know the parameters of the distribution you are measuring, and so the effect size cannot be calculated. However, if you perform a pilot study, the parameters may be estimated from the pilot study results. Alternatively, you may use Cohen's definitions of large, medium and small effect sizes, electing to design a study with a sample size that will detect (for a given power, usually 0.8) a small, medium or large effect.

Cohen[1] gives tables for:

- Student's *t*-test
- Pearson's correlation coefficient
- sign test
- chi square (χ^2) test
- *F* test (analysis of variance)
- Regression analysis.

In this chapter we give examples of the first four, as these are such common statistical tests in health research, and it is quite simple to perform a power analysis on them. For the last two items you are referred to Cohen.[1]

Example

I want to know whether there is a difference in the marks obtained by two successive cohorts of students. I know from previous years that the standard deviation of this examination is about 5.0. I am interested in detecting a difference of more than two percentage points, as I am not concerned (or, more importantly, my external examiners will accept such variability) if successive years differ by less than 2% even if the difference is statistically significant, as such a difference is not likely in practice to affect a student's overall degree grade. I want to use the conventional value $\alpha = 0.05$.

Cohen defines effect in this context (Student's t-test) as being the z score, i.e. the difference between the means divided by the standard deviation.[7] Thus I am looking to detect an effect of 2.0/5.0 or 0.4. Suppose I elect for a power of 0.8. Look at the power table for Student's t-test with $\alpha = 0.05$,[8] a portion of which is shown in Table 12.1, where the effect is denoted by d, and the critical value of d is considered to be when the power is 0.5, and is denoted by d_c. A graph based on these data is shown in Figure 12.1, which may be used to interpolate some points

Table 12.1 Power table for Student's unrelated (independent groups) t-test with sample size (n) for different effect sizes (d) at an α level of 0.05

n	d_c	d 0.10	0.20	0.30	0.40	0.50	0.60	0.70	0.80	1.00	1.20	1.40
10	0.78	0.08	0.11	0.16	0.22	0.29	0.36	0.45	0.53	0.70	0.83	0.91
13	0.67	0.08	0.13	0.18	0.26	**0.34**	0.44	0.54	**0.63**	0.80	0.91	0.97
20	0.53	0.09	0.15	0.24	0.34	0.46	0.59	0.70	0.80	0.93	0.98	
30	0.43	0.10	0.19	0.31	0.46	0.61	0.74	0.85	0.92	0.99		
40	0.37	0.11	0.22	0.38	0.55	0.72	0.84	0.93	0.97			
60	0.30	0.13	0.29	0.50	0.70	0.86	0.95	0.98				
80	0.26	0.15	0.35	0.60	**0.81**	0.93	0.98					
100	0.23	0.17	0.41	0.68	0.88	0.97						
200	0.16	0.26	0.64	0.91	0.99							

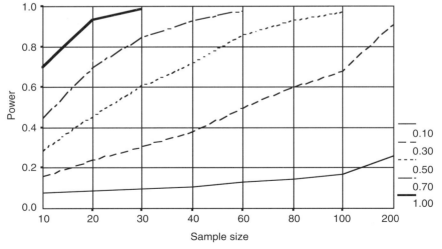

Figure 12.1 Student's t-test: Power for various effect magnitudes and sample sizes, using an alpha value of 0.05.

that are missing. (All the tables and graphs in this chapter are based on Cohen's text),[1] although he gives much fuller tables and tables for many more α levels and degrees of freedom (where appropriate, in χ^2 for example). While only a selection of values is given here, some of the intervening values of particular relevance to this text are given.) Thus as $d = 0.4$ and the power is 0.8 (shown in bold), which indicates that I will have to sample about 80 students.

Example

I want to check whether students in the child health branch are performing better or worse than students in the adult branches in their final degree marks. There are only 10 students in the child health branch, but there are 20 in the adult health branch. I want to know the power of detecting a medium effect size difference ($d = 0.5$).

As the groups are of unequal size, I need to adjust n. The formula for doing this is[9]

$$n' \frac{2n_a n_b}{n_a + n_b}$$

where n' is called the *harmonic mean*, and may be used in place of n when the two group sizes differ. If our case,

$$n' = \frac{2 \times 10 \times 20}{30} \simeq 13$$

The power is somewhere between 0.29 ($n = 10$) and 0.46 ($n = 20$). In fact from Cohen's tables for $n = 13$ it is 0.34 (shown in bold in Table 12.1). Thus there is only a moderate probability of noting even a moderate effect, and about two times in three we would miss it with these numbers. However, a large effect ($d = 0.8$) would be seen more readily with a power of between 0.53 ($n = 10$) and 0.80 ($n = 20$), and in fact from Cohen's tables for $n = 13$ the effect is given as 0.63 (shown in bold in Table 12.1). Thus roughly two-thirds of the time we would expect to detect a large effect.

Example

In a pilot study of computer network usage[10] 50 health trusts were approached and asked (among other things) if they had training on networked computing systems for nurses. A total of 21 replied, of which 15 were in England, and two each were in the other three countries, of the UK. The data split by country for England and Scotland shown in Table 12.2. (Data was also collected on Northern Ireland and Wales, but for simplicity we concentrate on only two countries in this example.)

Table 12.2 The number of health trusts in England and Scotland with computer training for nurses

Country	Training	No training	Total
England	7	8	15
Scotland	2	0	2
Total	9	8	17

Superficially it appears that England is worse at providing training, as about half the English sites give training, while both the Scottish sites do. However, the numbers are so small that using the χ^2 test at all is dubious (see Ch. 5), although the use of χ^2 with Yate's correction may be recommended and this gives a χ^2 value of 0.443, with $p = 0.51$. (Fisher's test, which might be considered appropriate, gives $p = 0.26$.) So although both the Scottish sites give training, the result is still not significant, either χ^2 corrected for continuity or with Fisher's exact test. The sample size is too small to make any meaningful statement about this result. What might we expect if we sample all trusts?

The effect size for a χ^2 of i cells is given by Cohen[1] as:

$$w = \sqrt{\frac{\sum(P_{1i} - P_{0i})^2}{P_{0i}}}$$

where P_{1i} is the proportion of cells expected (i.e. that predicted by the null hypothesis) and P_{0i} is the proportion of cells observed. We can re-jig the table to give the values (all rounded to two places of decimals) shown in Table 12.3. The expected values for proportions under the null hypothesis are given in Table 12.4.

Thus the effect size is

Table 12.3 Actual ratios

Country	Training	No training	Country marginal
England	0.41	0.47	0.88
Scotland	0.12	0.00	0.12
Training marginal	0.53	0.47	1.0

Table 12.4 Expected ratios

Country	Training	No training	Country marginal
England	0.47	0.41	0.88
Scotland	0.06	0.06	0.12
Training marginal	0.53	0.47	1.0

$$w = \sqrt{(0.41 - 0.47)^2 + (0.47 - 0.41)^2 + (0.12 - 0.06)^2 + (0.00 - 0.06)^2}$$
$$= \sqrt{0.14}$$
$$= 0.38$$

Thus we have a medium to large effect (Cohen[11] defines $w = 0.1$ to be small, $w = 0.3$ medium, and $w = 0.5$ a large effect. Therefore, paradoxically, we have a large effect being seen as not significant, which must be because we have an insufficient sample size.

Cohen gives tables for χ^2, and a selection of values from the table for $\alpha = 0.01$ and one degree of freedom[12] is given in Table 12.5. Thus we would have needed a sample size of somewhere between 50 and a 100 to detect even a large effect of $w = 0.5$ with a power of 0.5, i.e. to get a significant result 50% of the time when a real effect exists (in fact we would need a sample of about 75).

However, 0.01 is a very conservative value of α, and the more conventional value of 0.05 would give the effect sizes and powers shown in Table 12.6 and Figure 12.2. So using the more conventional α value gives a power of 0.7 for a large effect for a sample size of 25 (the lowest Cohen offers, which should give an indication that we are being optimistic using a sample as small as 17). This means that with a slightly larger sample than we have used, about one-third of the time we will miss even a large effect, even with $\alpha = 0.05$.

Table 12.5   Power table for the χ^2 test (one degree of freedom) with sample size (n) for different effect sizes (w) at an α level of 0.01, and with one degree of freedom

n	w 0.10	0.20	0.30	0.40	0.50	0.60	0.70	0.80	1.00
25	0.01	0.02	0.03	0.05	0.09	0.16	0.27	0.41	0.57
50	0.01	0.02	0.06	0.13	0.27	0.48	0.70	0.87	0.96
100	0.02	0.05	0.16	0.41	0.72	0.92	0.99		
200	0.02	0.13	0.48	0.87	0.99				
500	0.07	0.56	0.98						

Table 12.6   Power table for the χ^2 test (one degree of freedom) with sample size (n) for different effect sizes (w) at an α level of 0.05

n	w 0.10	0.20	0.30	0.40	0.50	0.60	0.70	0.80	1.00
25	0.08	0.17	0.32	0.52	0.70	0.85	0.94	0.98	0.99
50	0.11	0.29	0.56	0.81	0.94	0.99			
100	0.17	0.52	0.85	0.98					
200	0.29	0.81	0.99						
250	**0.35**	**0.89**							
⋮									
500	0.61	0.99							

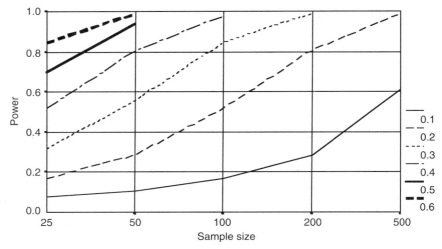

Figure 12.2 Chi square: Power for various effect magnitudes and sample sizes, using an alpha value of 0.05 and one degree of freedom.

Suppose we now want to estimate the power of our larger sample. We want to sample all the relevant health trusts in the UK, which when the survey was done was 355. If all trusts responded (unlikely) we would have a power of between 0.29 ($n = 200$) and 0.61 ($n = 500$) for a small effect ($w = 0.1$). In fact the nearest figure for $n = 350$ is 0.46, so even a small effect would be picked up about half (46%) of the time, and for $n = 350$ an effect of $w = 0.2$ is detected with a power of 0.96, (i.e. almost always).

In practice, about 73% of the health trusts responded after a letter and a reminder (similar figures responding to both). Do we need to worry about the response rate? On comparing the responses to the first and second tranch of replies no significant differences were noted, so it is reasonable to assume that the responses were representative. As the second tranch of responders were non-responders to the first letter, it would seem that non-responders are similar to responders when they are prompted to reply. Furthermore, even if the remaining 28% of health trusts were totally unlike the responders (unlikely), we still have a large proportion of the population, so that at the very least we can say about four-fifths of the trusts show certain characteristics. So we are left with the problem of the sample size.

The response was $n = 259$ which from Cohen's table for $n = 250$ (see Table 12.6) gives a power of 0.35 and 0.89 (shown in bold) for $w = 0.1$ and $w = 0.2$ respectively at $\alpha = 0.05$. So we have a one in three chance of detecting a small effect, and a nine in ten chance of detecting a small to moderate effect. In fact no significant differences were noted when all the trusts were analysed, leading us to the conclusion that the large effect noted in the pilot study was an artefact caused by an insufficient sample size.

Example

In a correlation test the serum albumin level is to be correlated with a nutrition assessment tool, the data provided by which have been found to be normally distributed (this is a fictional example, but such assessment tools do exist). To detect a small, medium or large effect how many patients would need to be assessed at $\alpha = 0.05$ and a power of 0.8?

To determine this consider the data given in Table 12.7 and Figure 12.3. According to Cohen,[13] a small effect is a correlation of $r = 0.1$, a medium effect one of $r = 0.3$ and a large effect one of $r = 0.5$. So for $r = 0.1$ a power of 0.8 is seen to give a sample size of somewhere between 100 and 1000, in fact it is at about 600

Table 12.7 Pearson correlation coefficient (r): effect magnitudes (correlation coefficients) and sample sizes, using an α value of 0.05

		r								
n	r_c	0.10	0.20	0.30	0.40	0.50	0.60	0.70	0.80	1.00
10	0.549	0.08	0.14	0.22	0.32	0.46	0.62	0.79	0.93	0.99
20	0.378	0.11	0.22	0.37	0.56	0.75	0.90	0.98		
23	0.352	0.12	0.24	0.41	0.62	**0.81**	0.94	0.99		
30	0.306	0.13	0.28	0.50	0.72	0.90	0.98			
40	0.264	0.15	0.35	0.60	0.83	0.96				
50	0.235	0.17	0.41	0.69	0.90	0.98				
68	0.201	0.20	0.50	**0.81**	0.96					
100	0.165	0.26	0.64	0.92	0.99					
600	0.067	**0.79**								
1000	0.052	0.96								

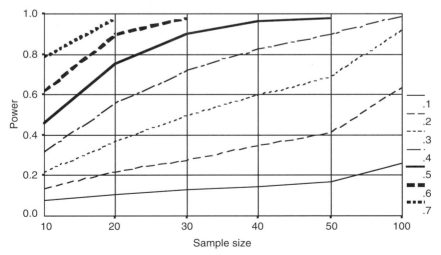

Figure 12.3 Pearson correlation coefficient: effect magnitudes (correlation coefficients) and sample sizes, using an alpha value of 0.05.

(shown in bold). For $r = 0.3$, a sample size of 50–100 would suffice (in fact 68 would work; value shown in bold) and for $r = 0.5$ a sample of only 23 suffices (shown in bold).

Example

In an assessment of pressure sores, staff are asked to note whether a sore is better, worse or the same as on a previous occasion. The sign test would be an appropriate test.

Cohen defines the effect in the sign test[14] as being the discrepancy in the proportions that are positive and negative. A null effect, where 50% are positive and 50% negative (equivalently, a ratio of 0.5 : 0.5) would have an effect of zero, as expected. Other values are given by the effect g, defined as the difference between the ratios found and 0.5:

Small effect $g = 0.05 \, (0.55 : 0.45)$
Medium effect $g = 0.15 \, (0.65 : 0.35)$
Large effect $g = 0.25 \, (0.75 : 0.25)$

Therefore, in order to note a small change, Table 12.8 (see also Fig. 12.4) shows us that for $\alpha = 0.05$ and a power of 0.8 we will need nearer to 1000 subjects than 100. In fact around 600 subjects (shown in bold in the table) would be sufficient to note a small change. To see a medium effect, between 50 and 100 subjects (in fact 64 would suffice; shown in bold) would be needed, and for a large effect we would need only about 20 subjects (in fact 21 is nearer the mark; shown in bold).

CONCLUSION

Sample sizes can be estimated either for descriptive studies or inferential studies. In the former, the parameters of the population need to be known

Table 12.8 Sign test: effect of magnitudes and sample sizes (n) using an α value of 0.05

n	a_1	w 0.05	0.10	0.15	1/6	0.20	0.25	0.30	0.35	0.40
10	0.055	0.10	0.17	0.26	0.30	0.38	0.53	0.68	0.82	0.93
20	0.058	0.13	0.25	0.42	0.48	0.61	0.74	0.91	0.98	
21	0.039	0.10	0.20	0.36	0.42	0.55	**0.79**	0.89	0.97	
30	0.049	0.14	0.29	0.51	0.58	0.73	0.89	0.97		
40	0.040	0.13	0.32	0.57	0.66	0.81	0.95	0.99		
50	0.059	0.20	0.45	0.73	0.80	0.92	0.99			
64	0.052	0.20	0.49	**0.79**	0.86	0.95				
100	0.044	0.24	0.62	0.91	0.96	0.99				
600	0.047	**0.78**								
⋮										
1000	0.047	0.93								

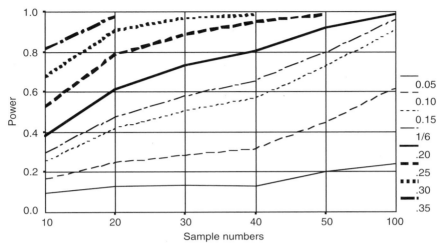

Figure 12.4 Sign test: effect magnitudes and sample sizes, using an alpha value of 0.05.

or estimated. In the latter case an effect size needs to be known, or the definitions used for small, medium or large effects may be used. In clinical practice the clinically significant effect may be estimated, and used to predict the sample size required to detect an effect that is meaningful for a given power.

The use of power analysis will reduce the likelihood of false inferences being made from inadequate sample sizes, and focus our attention on practically meaningful results, rather than statistically significant results. The latter are necessary, but are not in themselves meaningful unless accompanied by clinically significant outcomes.

EXERCISES

1. A (fictional) Pearson's correlation test for anxiety against salary gave $r = -0.1$ and $p = 0.01$. Comment on the statistical and clinical significance.
2. How large a sample would I need to detect an effect size of 0.3 for two equally sized groups using the independent groups Student's t-test, with a power of 0.8?

REFERENCES

1. Cohen J 1977 Statistical power analysis for the behavioral sciences. Academic Press, New York
2. Stuart A 1984 The ideas of sampling. Charles Griffin, High Wycombe
3. Cohen J 1977 Statistical power analysis for the behavioral sciences. Academic Press, New York, p 79–81

4. Cohen J 1977 Statistical power analysis for the behavioral sciences. Academic Press, New York, p 109–144
5. Chatfield C 1978 Statistics for technology. Chapman & Hall, London, p 158–163
6. Cohen J 1977 Statistical power analysis for the behavioral sciences. Academic Press, New York, p 56
7. Cohen J 1977 Statistical power analysis for the behavioral sciences. Academic Press, New York, p 21
8. Cohen J 1977 Statistical power analysis for the behavioral sciences. Academic Press, New York, p 30–31
9. Cohen J 1977 Statistical power analysis for the behavioral sciences. Academic Press, New York, p 43
10. Anthony D M 1997 A comparative study of computer networks in the NHS and the academic sector of the UK. Nursing Standard 11(18): 34–38
11. Cohen J 1977 Statistical power analysis for the behavioral sciences. Academic Press, New York, p 224–225
12. Cohen J 1977 Statistical power analysis for the behavioral sciences. Academic Press, New York, p 235
13. Cohen J 1977 Statistical power analysis for the behavioral sciences. Academic Press, New York, p 79–81
14. Cohen J 1977 Statistical power analysis for the behavioral sciences. Academic Press, New York, p 151

13

Errors in the use of statistics

Many journals show statistical error, even those that have been peer reviewed. The errors seen are in many cases elementary, and can cast doubt on the credibility of the work. Problems have been documented in the best medical journals, as well as nursing and journals devoted to PAM. This chapter discusses some of the more common misconceptions, errors and reporting failures, and offers a check list to ensure your study does not include the more common errors.

KEY POINTS

- Journal articles frequently contain errors in the reporting of statistics

- Most statistics errors are those of omission, where information is missing

- You should employ a check-list similar to the one at the end of this chapter when writing your study, or reviewing another author's study

At the end of this chapter the student should be able to:

1. Critically assess the statistics content of research articles
2. Design a study with appropriate statistical methods

INTRODUCTION

Statistics are very frequently used in research articles. It is commonly assumed, falsely, that a research article has to have a statistical basis. Where statistics are employed they are frequently used incorrectly, or insufficient detail is given to assure the reader that the statistics have been properly addressed. There have been many reviews of statistical methods in medical journals, which have shown that both the understanding of statistics and the reporting of the results is flawed in even the best peer-reviewed journals. The studies show that error rates upwards of 45% may be expected in high-quality mainstream refereed medical journals. While many of these errors are trivial, and often errors of omission, nonetheless they take credibility away from papers that are otherwise typically both relevant to the subject and theoretically sound.

For example, Gore et al[1] examined 77 reports in the *British Medical Journal* that contained numerical analysis. Of these 81% contained statistical analysis. They found that 52% of the reports with statistical analysis included at least one error and 8% made a claim in the summary that was not supported by the data. White[2] looked at 168 papers from the *British Journal of Psychiatry* that contained numerical results, and found that 45% contained statistical errors. MacArthur & Jackson[3] examined 90 articles in the *Journal of Infectious Diseases*, of which 71% used statistical analysis; only 28% were considered to be error free.

Kanter & Taylor[4] looked at 122 papers in *Transfusion*, of which 48% contained statistical methods. Of these 39% contained an error in describing the statistical tests, 80% failed to describe clearly the tests employed, 75% used an incorrect test or contained an error in calculation or interpretation, and 22% gave conclusions that were not supported by the data. As Altman[5] points out, there is not merely an academic concern when statistical analyses are not carried out properly, as ethical issues are raised where practice is based on spurious results.

The concern shown by the medical press about statistics errors in articles led me to explore the nursing press, where I expected at least as gloomy a picture. I chose to look at the *Journal of Advanced Nursing*, a well-respected international academic nursing journal. If this journal showed similar problems as the medical press, we could expect even worse cases in the journals showing less academic rigour. The results were reported in the *Journal of Advanced Nursing*.[6]

Comparing 1986 with 1996, the percentages of papers containing statistical analysis remained remarkably constant. Just over one-half of the papers were not quantitative in nature, and of the remaining quantitative papers about one-half gave descriptive statistics only, with the other half (30% of the total papers) having some form of statistical analysis. The articles were analysed for the occurrence of several common errors noted in previous reviews of medical journals. The nursing articles were comparable with those in medical journals with respect to the overall percentage of errors noted, although the types of error encountered were slightly different, but explicable by the different types of data that nurses use. In particular, nursing studies are far less likely to involve the use of interval/ratio scales. Accordingly, they were more prone to use parametric tests on data not shown to be normally distributed.

This chapter now looks at the typical errors found in the literature, as shown in the studies above, and describes in more detail both the errors and how to avoid them.

DEFINING THE STUDY

Sample size

Inferential tests completed on too small a sample will give excessive type II errors. While it is difficult to state in advance the sample size needed in all cases, there are tables you can consult that give sample sizes for given tests and given power.

Random selection

If inferential tests are being completed, then the results will be meaningless unless the samples have been selected appropriately, this usually involving some form of random selection.

Hypotheses and research questions

One of the most common mistakes I see in research theses is the absence of a research question or hypothesis. Any research should have clear aim and objectives. Typically, these may be framed in the form of one or more questions that are to be answered. A research question is typically used in qualitative or descriptive quantitative studies. In inferential statistics you need one or more hypotheses.

The research question or hypothesis allows you to determine whether you have met the aims of the study, either by answering a question or by accepting or rejecting a hypothesis. Conventionally, the null hypothesis is given. For example:

Null hypothesis: There is no significant difference in attitude to complementary therapies between the first and fourth year students in a physiotherapy degree.

as opposed to the experimental hypothesis

Experimental hypothesis: There is a significantly more favourable attitude to complementary therapies by fourth year students in a physiotherapy degree than by the first year students.

The reason for giving the null hypothesis is that the experimental hypothesis would be rejected if the first year students had a more favourable attitude, or if they were the same with respect to attitude. Using a null hypothesis allows you to explore the direction of the difference once you have identified a difference exists (i.e. it is two-tailed rather than one-tailed).

If a hypothesis is given it should be absolutely clear and unambiguous. A common problem is to merge several hypotheses together. For example:

Hypothesis: There is no significant difference in knowledge of and attitude to complementary therapies between the first and fourth year students in a physiotherapy degree.

In the above hypothesis you would have to reject the (null) hypothesis if either knowledge *or* attitude were different. The null hypothesis is accepted therefore if knowledge is significantly different and attitude is not, or if attitude is significantly different and knowledge is not. Furthermore changing the 'and' to 'or' makes a big difference to interpreting the result of the test, as now the null hypothesis is accepted only if *neither* attitude nor knowledge is significantly different. The hypothesis is not sufficiently specific. It is much preferred to have two hypotheses:

Hypothesis 1: There is no significant difference in knowledge of complementary therapies between the first and fourth year students in a physiotherapy degree.

Hypothesis 2: There is no significant difference in attitude to complementary therapies between the first and fourth year students in a physiotherapy degree.

DESCRIPTION OF DATA

Dispersion

If you have normally distributed data, then quoting the mean and standard deviation will give the reader a precise description of the distribution. If, however, the distribution of the data is not normal, these values are all but meaningless.

For non-normal data the median or mode is typically a better measure of central tendency than the mean. Since the measures of central tendency tell us different things about a non-normal distribution, all three measures (mean, mode and median) may be used to describe central tendency in a non-normal distribution.

There are ways of describing the distribution of values of non-normal data. For example, the range, inter-quartile range, or some percentile points, say the 5th to 95th percentile, can be used to describe the variability of the data. However, there are no definitive parameters that succinctly describe most non-normal distributions, and a simple histogram or table of frequencies is often the best way of showing the distribution.

If the distribution is normal, then about 95% of the data will lie within two standard deviations of the mean. It is a common convention to show the mean and two standard deviations as a measure of the range. For example, if the mean pulse rate of a sample were 70 beats per minute with a standard deviation of 5 beats per minute, then 70.0 ± 10.0 might be used to describe the range of 95% of the data. However, it is also common to show the range as the mean $\pm$ one standard deviation, so unless the description is made explicit the reader does not know the range with certainty.

A further problem arises as many authors use the standard error of the mean (SEM) rather than the standard deviation. The SEM is typically used incorrectly. The use of the SEM rather than the standard deviation is a common but incorrect method of describing data distribution.[7] Reasons for using the SEM include tradition and the fact that it is always smaller than the standard deviation. The SEM describes the variability of the mean for several samples drawn from the same population. Therefore it may be used to state within what range the mean values typically lie, so 95% of the means will be within two SEMs. In other words the SEM does not measure the dispersion of a sample; rather, it is a measure of the certainty that the sample mean estimates the population mean.[3] It is not appropriate to use the SEM as a measure of spread for the distribution; you should use the standard deviation for that purpose.

Studies have shown that 31% of papers in the *Journal of Infectious Diseases* misused the SEM[3] and 39% of the papers in *Transfusion*[4] showed this error. Since the SEM is so frequently used in error where the standard deviation should be used, and since it is often not clear how many standard deviations are being quoted in a range, you should be totally explicit when using the '$\pm$' notation.

The study of articles in the *Journal of Advanced Nursing*,[6] 13% used the mean alone or the mean and standard deviation with non-normal data, and 11% misused the '±' notation. If your data are not known to be normal, do not use the standard deviation as your sole measure of dispersion, and if your data are normal (which usually implies they are interval/ratio level data) specify the number of standard deviations used in defining a range.

Rounding of numbers

Two concepts are important here: precision and accuracy.[8] If a measurement is taken several times then it does not, in general, give exactly the same result, as there may be errors involved in the recording. There may be variations due to the changing environmental conditions of laboratory equipment (e.g. room temperature may change) or errors may be caused by human variability (e.g. the investigator is more tired the second time, and takes less care in the measurement). The degree to which a measurement is repeatable is the *precision*. A high precision means that the recorded value varies only slightly, which in a normal distribution would mean a small standard deviation.

However, a high precision does not imply high *accuracy*, which is a measure of how free from bias the measurement is. For example, a blood glucose test may give a very similar result every time, but always be about 2 mmol/l from the true value. Another machine may give less precise but more accurate readings. An inaccurate but precise measurement indicates a lack of calibration, i.e. the measurement should be adjusted to coincide with the true value.

It is very misleading to state, for example, the blood glucose measurement from a machine that is only precise to one place of decimals was 4.4636 mmol/l. It is better to round values to appropriate figures, here to 4.5 mmol/l.

It is also not helpful to quote very high precision on percentages where the numbers involved are small. For example, if three of nine people in a sample are black, stating that 33.3333% are black is misleading, and even 33% in this case might imply a level of confidence we do not possess. Where numbers are very small and percentages are given, especially where they are used for comparison with other figures, the actual numbers should be given as well.

Finally, you should have some measure of how well the measuring device is performing with respect to accuracy. Quoting a highly precise measurement that is wholly inaccurate is clearly not appropriate. This is typically the more difficult aspect to address, as you may not know the true value, or the measurement made is your best method of finding the true value. Consider the example of diagnosis of distal fracture from radiographs that we looked at in Chapter 8. The gold standard was the opinion of a consultant radiologist. But how would we measure the consultant's accuracy? Another example is that of measuring poverty. An economist might present precise figures for income, but if income is not the only or the best measure of poverty (there are other variables, e.g. family support, level of dependence by others, area of habitation and access to cheap shopping) this may be misleading. Hence the cliché that an economist prefers to be precisely wrong than roughly right.

DESCRIPTION OF STATISTICAL TESTS
Significance

You will often see comments such as 'a significant difference was seen', but with no mention of what test was used to determine the significance of the result. Alternatively, where more than one test is possible, for example with correlation, the test actually used is often not identified. Since, where there is a choice of tests, one is typically parametric and the other non-parametric, failure to specify the test makes it impossible to ascertain whether the statistical approach is correct or optimal. In some studies several tests are used, but it is not made clear which test is used on which data.

MacArthur & Jackson[3] showed that 27% of articles in the *Journal of Infectious Diseases* failed to identify correctly at least one of the tests performed, and Kanter & Taylor[4] showed that 13% of the papers with statistical analysis published in *Transfusion* failed to state the statistical test used. In the study of papers in the *Journal of Advanced Nursing*,[6] 18% of the studies failed to state the statistical test employed. In six of the eight cases a correlation test was employed, which could have been one of several, though typically the Pearson or Spearman rank tests are used. However, the assumptions are different for the Pearson and the Spearman tests (Pearson, assuming normality of data, is a parametric test; Spearman is a non-parametric test) and thus knowledge of the test used is necessary. In addition, where more than one test was used in a study, 7% failed to identify which test was used on which data.[6]

The p value is a number that ranges between zero and one; mathematically this is denoted by [0.0,1.0]. The p value is the probability of getting the results by chance alone. A low p value shows that the results are unlikely to have occurred by chance, while a high p value indicates that is quite plausible that the results are explicable by chance (i.e. random) fluctuations in the data. However unlikely it is that data could have occurred by chance, there is always a finite possibility that this is the case. While it may be more likely that I will win the pools (which I enter each week in preference to the lottery) than that the data I obtained was by chance alone, it is still possible, however remote such a possibility may be.

SPSS (and other statistics packages) reports a p value to a designated number of decimal places, typically three or four. So a result of one in a million ($p = 0.000001$) could not be shown, as it needs six decimal places. It is thus rounded to the nearest figure that SPSS can show, which in this case, if four decimal places are shown, is $p = 0.0000$. This indicates a p value of exactly zero, which is impossible. If you see such a value, all you can say is that, as four decimal places cannot show the exact value, it must be $p < 0.0001$, which is how you must describe the result. I have seen many student dissertations and some published papers that contain the elementary error of quoting a p value of zero. This presumably occurs as the author copies (or pastes) the result directly from the statistics package to the word processor. This type of error suggests you are using a statistics package with a shallow knowledge of statistics, and casts doubt on the statistics used in the paper.

Failure to define details of test

There are four very common errors in reporting the output of a test:

Failure to state whether a test is one- or two-tailed

Is the test one-tailed or two-tailed? In the vast majority of cases a two-tailed test is the more appropriate. If you were testing the significance of the difference between the mean values for two groups A and B for some variable (pulse rate, say), you should only use a one-tailed test if one group is expected to have the higher mean value (say group A) and it is impossible or uninteresting if group B turns out to have the higher mean value. Such cases are rare, and it is assumed that any test that is not stated to be one-tailed is in fact two-tailed. Unfortunately, it is not unknown for a researcher to perform a test, note that it just fails to reach significance, and repeat the test as a one-tailed test, where it now reaches significance. To guard against this error it helps if the precise test is stated, and on the rare occasions where a one-tailed test is appropriate the rationale given clearly. If you see a one-tailed test performed without any credible rationale you should treat the result with caution. One general exception to this rule is the use of Fisher's exact test. In the most common use of Fisher's test we are interested in whether we could have got by chance the number of cases observed or less; this situation is inherently one-tailed. In the *Journal of Advanced Nursing*,[6] 83% of studies that used a test that could be one- or two-tailed (Student's t-test, Pearson, etc.) failed to state which version of the test was employed.

Failure to state whether a test is paired or unpaired

Some tests are inherently unpaired (e.g. Mann–Whitney) and some are always used with paired data (e.g. Wilcoxon). But others (e.g. Student's *t*-test) come in both paired and unpaired versions. Some authors use the wrong version of Student's *t*-test, and the results of, for example, the paired test on unpaired data will be meaningless. Therefore you should always state which version of a test you have used if there is more than one. In the papers from the *Journal of Advanced Nursing*,[6] 20% failed to state whether a test was paired or unpaired, when either version was a possibility.

Failure to state which version of a test is used

For some tests there is more than one way of computing the result. In many cases corrections are made to the test statistic to allow for departure from the assumptions of the test. Chi square (χ^2) is an example of a test that can generate several different results, depending on whether various corrections are made. It is advised, if the size of the samples is small, that Yate's continuity correction is used; if the sample is large, using Yate's correction does not affect the result much anyway, so some writers advise its use routinely. As the output from small samples can be affected by the use of Yate's correction, you should state whether it has been used. Of the studies reported in the *Journal of Advanced Nursing*[6] that used the χ^2 test, none stated whether the Yate's correction was used. Another example is the independent-groups Student's *t*-test, which assumes equal variance in the two groups. But allowance can be made for the situation where variance is not equal. In SPSS the independent-groups Student's *t*-test checks for equal variance, and gives a correction for unequal variance by adjusting the degrees of freedom of the test. As the variance of the two groups diverge, the two results also become quite different.

Failure to define the α level

There is a convention that the α level, the probability below which the null hypothesis is to be rejected, is set at 0.05. However, this is only a convention, and from time to time you will see α levels set at, for example, 0.1. I am always a bit suspicious when I see such an α level, as it may be set after the result was obtained, and found to be above 0.05. But some writers do recommend the use of different α levels for different sample sizes in order to avoid excessive type II errors in very small samples. Therefore you should always state the level at which a value is to be considered significant, and not simply remark that a result is significant. In the *Journal of Advanced Nursing* study,[6] the α level was not explicitly set in 76% of the studies.

USE OF A STATISTICAL TEST
Do we need inferential tests?

I frequently discuss study designs with students who want to know what tests they need to use. In many cases the answer is none. Simply performing inferential tests because they are available and can be used on your data is not advisable. Having stated your research question, which may or may not have an associated hypothesis, you next need to establish how to address that question. If a quantitative study is purely descriptive then the research question is answered directly by the results.

Some studies consist of or contain qualitative data, which are not (usually) amenable to statistical analysis other than tabulating responses after content analysis. For example, in my study of the use of computer networks in health trusts and academic organizations, I asked:[9]

Please state any views you may have on the use or potential use of large national/international computer networks to assist nurses/midwives in providing and improving patient care.

This is too loosely structured to be amenable to statistical analysis. However, this is not a criticism, simply a comment. To give a more structured question I would have needed to know the possible answers, which at the time I did not have. This is a classic use of qualitative analysis, i.e. to explore a subject with open questions, possibly to allow future closed questions after content analysis.

However, when I wanted to know in how many health trusts nurses had access to computer networks,[9] then the answer was obtained by descriptive statistics, in this case a raw number of trusts or a percentage of trusts. Some of the research questions were:

- What computer network resources are available?
- Do trusts and other organizations access the networks and, if so, how?

The answers to these questions are obtained by identifying and counting the resources, and by counting the trusts and other organizations that access networks, and by tabulating and counting the methods of access. No inferential test is relevant to address these particular questions.

There were questions in the study that did need inferential tests (e.g. Is there a difference between the different types of organizations in their access to networks?), and one hypothesis might be:

There is no significant difference in Internet access between health trusts and academic sites.

A hypothesis needs some method of assessment to determine whether to accept or reject the hypothesis, which is typically an inferential test. Here the χ^2 test could be used.

A general rule is that if your research question can be put in the form of a hypothesis then you should look to an inferential test. If your research question is answered by a description of the data then it is unlikely that an inferential test will be helpful. If your data are obtained from unstructured interviews, focus groups or open questions in a questionnaire, then there is limited utility in calculating even descriptive statistical parameters. What is most useful in such data is the generation of theories, not of (probably meaningless) numbers. Some studies only require descriptive statistical methods, while others are purely qualitative. Many studies, like the one mentioned above, have both qualitative and quantitative data, and the latter may be addressed by both descriptive and inferential methods.

Incompatible or inappropriate tests

Apart from using parametric tests on non-normal data, which is inappropriate, and using non-parametric tests on normal data, which is often suboptimal, some authors simply use a test that cannot possibly perform the function of testing the hypothesis set. In 9% of the papers used tests that appeared to be incompatible with the type of data used.[6] These included:

● *Correlation on data that were nominal*. This might be acceptable if a contingency table was used to compute a correlation using Cramer's *V* (a correlation coefficient for two nominal scores based on χ^2), but from the context it was not obvious that this was done, and it is likely that a Pearson or Spearman rank analysis was computed. SPSS and other packages will let you do this, as it has no way of knowing that a nominal variable coded as a number is not, say, ordinal.

● χ^2 *on ordinal or interval data*. This is not strictly wrong, but is using a very weak test for ordinal/interval data.

● χ^2 *tests for independence of two variables*. If one variable is at the interval/ratio level and the other at the nominal level, ANOVA or an unrelated-variables Student's *t*-test (dependent on the number of groups in the nominal variable) would be much more powerful, and if the conditions of these tests did not apply then the equivalent non-parametric tests, Mann–Whitney or Kruskall–Wallis, should be used. If neither variable is nominal, χ^2 is an even more bizarre choice as the correlation tests (Pearson and Spearman rank) are available, although other tests may need to be considered if the relationship is non-linear.

Multiple pairwise comparisons

If you perform one test using an α level of 0.05, and it comes up with $p < 0.05$, then you reject the null hypothesis. But if you perform 20 similar tests in one batch, and one comes up at $p < 0.05$, while all the others are above the α level, the conclusion that the one result is significant is not acceptable, because you would expect one of the tests to give a type I error if the test were run on 20 data sets. There are methods of dealing with this situation; for example, you would use ANOVA to explore the difference among four groups, not perform six pairwise comparisons. If multiple testing is necessary then there are ways to calculate a new α level.

A major error in performing multiple pairwise comparisons is to under-estimate the α level required. Glantz[7] stated that a conservative estimate for the α value is obtained by adding the α values of each individual test together. Thus if three comparisons of three groups (A, B and C) are made (A versus B, B versus C and A versus C) a single quoted p value of < 0.05 equates to a $p < 0.15$. The use of the Bonferroni inequality (whereby the revised α level for a given single test for multiple comparisons is obtained by dividing the required α value by the number of comparisons) is recommended by MacArthur & Jackson,[3] although they note that it is too conservative a test if the number of pairwise comparisons is greater than five. Thus, while robust and unlikely to produce a type I error, the Bonferroni inequality is not very powerful and is quite likely to give a type II error as the number of pairwise comparisons increases. In general, there are better specific ways of dealing with most situations, for example analysis of variance (ANOVA) for independent groups (see Ch. 6).

In Anthony,[6] 44% of studies gave multiple pairwise comparisons, but did not account for the fact that multiple tests effect the α level. Despite the advice offered in the guidelines to contributors (e.g. Altman et al,[10] Murray[11] and Jamart[12]), failure to correct for multiple comparisons remains a common error. Kanter & Taylor[4] showed 22% of articles in *Transfusion* made this mistake, and this compares with 45% in the *Journal of Advanced Nursing*,[6] studies that were done very close together in time. This identi-fies an area where nursing studies seem to be particularly weak compared with medicine.

The question arises, then, of when several tests in a study require an altered α level. You might say that I need to adjust the level if I do, say, five tests in a paper, but no adjustment is needed if only one test is used. However, what would you say if I did five papers with one test in each using the same information? It would be rather strange if the α level depended on the brevity of a paper! To resolve this problem you should remember what it means to have a p value of 0.05. It means a type I error will occur roughly 5% of the time. Thus in 20 studies you would expect roughly one to give a false-positive result. It is on this basis that meta-analysis may be undertaken, where many studies are evaluated as a group. I would advise that if you are doing several tests that are all answer-ing different questions, or equivalently resolving different hypotheses, then no adjustment to the α levels is needed, but that from time to time a false-positive outcome will result (about 5% of the time). However, if multiple pairwise testing is undertaken to determine one hypothesis, then the α level will need adjustment.

Chi square on small samples

As shown in the chapter on contingency tables, when the expected value of a cell is below 5 in more than 20% of the cells, the output from the test is thought to be unreliable. It has been stated that Yate's correction gives results similar to Fisher's test, which would usually be the preferred test in such a circumstance.

Use of parametric tests on non-normal data

This is a particularly common error in health care research, as many of the data are not normally distributed, but many of the researchers have been trained in the use of parametric statistics. It is usually unnecessary to use parametric test on non-normal data as appropriate non-parametric tests are typically available. I have had arguments with both students and academic colleagues concerning the use of parametric tests on what I would consider inappropriate data, which in general means non-normal data, or data that are not shown to be normal, or could not be shown to be normal because of the level of granularity in the data. I have been told that the parametric tests are more powerful (which they are), that they are robust to departure from normality (which is true) and that the results are generally similar to those obtained using non-parametric tests (which is also often so).

However, I have a serious objection to this line of thought, based on two rather obvious observations:

- If two tests (one parametric and the other non-parametric) give the same results on a set of non-normal data, then there is no advantage in using the parametric test, other than that you may be more familiar with the parametric test (although how you will develop familiarity with non-parametric tests by using such an approach is unclear to me, and this seems a circular argument).
- If a parametric test gives a different result to a non-parametric test on non-normal data, why would we believe the test that makes assumptions that are not true rather than the test that makes no such false assumptions.

It seems to me that the philosophy of always using parametric tests is wrong, and based more on a desire to get a positive result rather than a valid one, or on familiarity of the investigator with the methods. It is true that on normal data a parametric test will (assuming the other conditions of the test are observed) make a type II error less likely that the corresponding non-parametric test, i.e. it is more powerful. Using a parametric test on data that are inappropriate will give more positive (apparently significant) results, but this is likely to be as a result of type I errors.

It seems to me that the only justification for using a parametric test on data it is not designed for is where no such non-parametric test exists, and then only in an exploratory fashion. Accordingly I have little problem with the use of factor analysis on non-normal data if it is used to generate a theory that is later tested. This is akin to using a qualitative methodology to develop a theory, and requires less rigour than true inferential testing.

In the *Journal of Advanced Nursing Study*,[6] 33% of studies used a parametric test on data that could not be assumed to be normal. These included Student's *t*-test, ANOVA, Pearson correlation and factor analysis using principal components analysis (PCA). (*Note*: It can be argued, as I have above, that as factor analysis is essentially a descriptive method, using it on non-normal data is not an error. However, the analysis does assume normality.)

While it is not always clear whether data are normal or not, give-away signs in an academic paper are:

- The mean, mode and median are very different (in a perfectly normal distribution they will be the same).
- Twice the standard deviation from the mean gives impossible values; for example, a serum level quoted as 5.0 with a standard deviation of 4.0. This gives a 95% range of 5.0 ± 8.0 or a range of $[-0.3, 13.0]$, and a negative serum level is clearly not possible.
- Visual inspection of the frequency histogram shows that the data are clearly skewed.
- An ordinal score with a low level of granularity is in use. Examination scores based on a percentage might be argued to be ordinal data, but found to be normally distributed. It is impossible even to check the normality of a Likert scale of four values.

There are tests for normality, such as the Kolmogorov–Smirnov goodness of fit test. However, few studies report the use of such a statistic. Parametric tests are robust to small departures from normality, and visual inspection of a histogram to check for approximate normality is acceptable.

One of the main abuses is incorrect use of Student's *t*-test. This is known to be a problematic area. In a study by Hall,[13] 71% of papers citing the *t*-test in the *British Journal of Surgery* in 1979 and 1980 were found to have made an error in using the test. In 15% of these cases an unpaired test was used on paired data, but the most common error was questionable normality of data, where 67% used the *t*-test on data that were probably not normally distributed. It should be added that health research outside of medicine (e.g. nursing) typically uses ordinal data, while medicine much more frequently employs interval/ratio data, which in addition could be normally distributed. Since nursing and other disciplines use data for which non-parametric tests may be more appropriate, workers in these areas should be aware of this potential problem.

ACCEPTANCE OF RESULTS
Approaching significance

I have seen academics of the highest calibre state that their results are almost significant, and that therefore when they have collected more data the results will be significant. This is not necessarily true and shows a complete misunderstanding of the statistical approach. If your tests approach but do not reach significance, then, at your given α level, the data you have do not support rejection of the null hypothesis. Obtaining more data might result in a significant finding, or the p value may actually increase. Adding more data makes you more confident either that there is or there is not an effect. It is not a unidirectional effect.

Not accepting the null hypothesis

Most researchers have an emotional commitment to their study. A statistical approach is designed to overcome this by giving a quantitative measure of the probability of getting a particular result. I have read dissertations that, having accepted the null hypothesis, then go on to discuss the reasons for a difference between two groups, or to account for a correlation. If you have found that your data could have occurred by chance alone, giving reasons other than chance to explain the data is worse than unnecessary.

It is so tempting to believe, typically on the basis of a small amount of data, that some apparent pattern or relationship in the data is meaningful, that special care needs to be taken. The use of inferential tests is in many cases that safeguard. You must accept the result of the test, rather than discount it and pretend it never happened. You are doing a statistical test to find out whether some pattern is meaningful, not to prove that it is. It is not a failure to find that a relationship between two variables is not supported by the data, a null result being as meaningful as a positive result. It simply means our original hunch (as stated in the hypothesis, albeit typically in the null form) is possibly wrong, and we should look for other explanations or theories.

It is of course true that there is always the possibility of a type II error, and all studies, whether showing positive or null results, are only to be considered our best guess given the current data. It is tempting to suggest, especially if the p value approaches significance, that additional data will show a significant result. This may be true, but the opposite might also occur, i.e. that additional data will confirm the null result. Having more data simply allows greater confidence in our results. I have seen eminent professors publicly make this elementary mistake, claiming that more data will show greater significance. Apart from being plain wrong, it begs the question of why did the researcher start with a sample size that they consider inadequate to answer the hypothesis? Either the sample size was inadequate, which indicates a design flaw, or it was sufficient, in which case we should accept the results.

We should mention here the difference between clinical and statistical significance. If in a large study a very small difference is noted, and found to be significant, this does not necessarily make it of practical importance. For example, a drug that reduced blood pressure by 0.1 mmHg is not of much use, even if it is known to a very high degree of certainty that it does in fact produce this reduction.

Not reporting null results

Related to the non-acceptance of the null hypothesis, is non-reporting of null results. A researcher may complete an experiment, find it gives no significant result, and then re-do the experiment several times until a positive result occurs. This is much more likely to happen in simulations or laboratory work than in survey or interview based research, as the possibility and cost of obtaining new samples is typically prohibitive in the latter. Repeating experiments until a positive (significant) result occurs is, of course, explicable by type I error, but this may not be obvious if the researcher simply publishes the significant results without mentioning the many nonsignificant trials.

This problem is not necessarily caused by the researcher. A study that shows no difference, or no relationship, or that a model does not work, is much less newsworthy than one that does. It is harder to get studies without a significant result into the academic press, and virtually impossible to get such studies into any other publication. Thus there is an inherent bias towards type I errors in the literature. You should not be surprised if the techniques showing such promise in published works fail to produce any benefit when you try them. When I was completing my doctoral studies I began to think I had the reverse Midas touch. I was trying several techniques, such as using genetic algorithms to create neural net designs (see Ch. 11) and altering the learning algorithm to accelerate learning in networks, and not one of them worked on my dataset, despite volumes of studies indicating how wonderful these techniques are on wide ranges of data. I suspect that the studies I read were somewhat selective in their reporting (this is not of course to say that the techniques do not work on the precise data/domains that they were reported to work on, simply that where they did not work it was difficult to get the studies published).

CONCLUSION

Most studies contain errors in definition of the statistics used, even if the tests are performed appropriately, and often that is not the case. Most studies in the scientific literature fail to identify an α level, and it is often implicit that the conventional level of $p < 0.05$ is in use. Similarly tests which may be one- or two-tailed, are usually assumed to be two-tailed unless otherwise stated. An explicit statement of the precise conditions and tests used avoids many potential misunderstandings.

Use of multiple pairwise comparisons with no adjustment of the alpha level is a more serious error as it raises type I errors. If 10 tests are made with, say, Student's t-test, then one would expect one of them to give $p < 0.05$ roughly half of the time, and not one time in 20 as might be reported.

CHECK-LIST

See that your analysis avoids the common problems discussed above by checking through the items below (adapted from Anthony[6]).

Defining the study

- Do you have an unambiguous research question or hypothesis? Have you merged more than one hypothesis together?

Sample

- Is your sample selected randomly?
- Is the sample large enough to perform statistical tests?

Improper description of data

- Have you used the ± notation without specifying whether it refers to standard deviation, standard error of the mean or some other measure of dispersion?
- Have you used the standard deviation as the sole measure of spread about the mean when the data are clearly not normal?
- Have you quoted values to unrealistic accuracy/precision?

Improper description of statistical tests

- Have you identified the statistical test performed? If you have used more than one type of statistical test is it clear when each test was used and on which data?
- Are you sure that the tests were performed on compatible data?
- Have you quoted an impossible p value ($p = 0.000$ for example)?
- Have you stated:
  - The number of tails (in Student's t-test, Pearson etc.)?
  - If Yate's correction was used in a χ^2 test?
  - Whether the test was paired or unpaired?
  - What values of p are significant (i.e. have you defined your α level)?

Improper use of a statistical test

- Do you need a test?

- Have you accounted for multiple pairwise comparisons?
- Have you used a χ^2 test on a contingency table when the expected frequency in more than 20% of the cells were less than 5?
- Have you used a paired test on unpaired data or an unpaired test on paired data?
- Have you used a parametric test on non-normal data? Have you checked for normality of your data?

Acceptance of results

- Have you ignored the result of inferential testing?
- Have you repeated the experiment, survey, etc., until you get a positive result?
- Have you moved on to a new area of study, not bothering to write up a null result?

REFERENCES

1. Gore S M, Jones I G, Rytter E C 1977 Misuse of statistical methods: Critical assessment of articles in *British Medical Journal* from January to March 1976. British Medical Journal 1: 85–87
2. White S J 1979 Statistical errors in papers in the *British Journal of Psychiatry*. British Journal of Psychiatry 135: 336–342
3. MacArthur R D, Jackson G G 1984 An evaluation of the use of statistical methods in the *Journal of Infectious Diseases*. Journal of Infectious Diseases 149(3): 349–354
4. Kanter M H, Taylor J R 1994 Accuracy of statistical methods in *Transfusion*: A review of articles from July/August 1992 through June 1993. Transfusion 34(8): 697–701
5. Altman D G 1980 Statistics and ethics in medical research: Misuse of statistics is unethical. British Medical Journal 281: 1182–1184
6. Anthony D M 1996 A review of statistical methods in the *Journal of Advanced Nursing*. Journal of Advanced Nursing 24: 1089–1094
7. Glantz S A 1980 Biostatistics: How to detect, correct and prevent errors in medical literature. Circulation 61(1): 1–7
8. Chatfield C 1978 Statistics for technology. Chapman & Hall, London, p 204
9. Anthony D M 1997 A comparative study of computer networks in the NHS and the academic sector of the UK. Nursing Standard 11(18): 34–38
10. Altman D G, Gore S M, Gardner M J, Pocock S J 1983 Statistical guidelines for contributors to medical journals. British Medical Journal 286: 1489–1494
11. Murray G D 1991 Statistical guidelines for the British Journal of Surgery. British Journal of Surgery 78: 782–784
12. Jamart J 1992 Statistical tests in medical research. Acta Oncologica 31(7): 723–727
13. Hall J C 1982 Use of the *t* test in the *British Journal of Surgery*. British Journal of Surgery 69: 55–56

Answers to exercises

Chapter 2: Introduction to SPSS

1. This will depend on your system, but for Windows '95 it will always be an option from the Start button. In the earlier versions of Windows one of the icons on the screen should be the SPSS icon; if this is not the case, then using Windows pull-down will allow you to locate it.

2. This is done simply by double clicking on the variable names at the top of the column, or using the Data pull-down and then selecting Define Variable. Just type in the variable name and then click on OK or hit the Enter key.

3. Simply type the values in the cells of each column.

4. Using the Define Variable method in (2) above, click on Type, and give zero decimal places (and, optionally, a length of one, as the variable is either 0 or 1).

5. Selecting Labels under Value Labels enter zero for Value and 'normal' for Value Label. Click on Add and do similar operation for the other value. Click on Continue, then OK.

6. Using Statistics, then Summarize and then Frequencies gives the following:

Value label	Frequency	%	%	%
0	6	54.5	54.5	54.5
1	5	45.5	45.5	100.0
Total	11	100.0	100.0	

Hence the answer is 5.

7. The pie chart will look as follows:

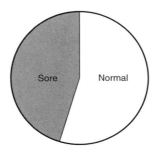

233

8. The histogram will look as follows:

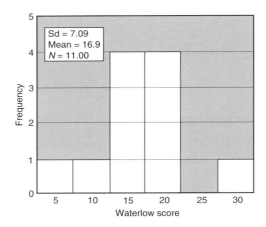

Chapter 3: Validity and reliability

1. Kappa is fair, according to Everitt and Landis & Koch, and the significance is very high (although not of course 0.00000, but $p < 0.00001$). Thus, while absolute agreement is not reached, this level of agreement is most unlikely to have occurred by chance.

2. We usually ask for an α value of over 0.7. Thus it would appear the components cannot be assumed to be measuring the same thing.

Chapter 4: Correlation and partial correlation

1. There is a significant ($p < 0.001$) negative correlation; i.e. as GDP increases, infant mortality goes down.

2. While GDP is likely to have a major effect on infant mortality, allowing for it does not remove the correlation between infant and perinatal mortality, so it would seem that the relationship is not (from this evidence) spurious.

Chapter 5: Contingency tables

1. Less men and more women have sores than you would expect. The significance is borderline, with Pearson's χ^2 being just under 0.05, and Yate's correction (Continuity correction) just above it. This shows that gender and presence of sores probably are not independent, but more data may be needed to establish one way or the other whether this dependency is real or a type I error.

2. Men (0) are about 37% more likely to be normal (no sores) and women about 21% less likely, but again the significance is marginal, as the value includes 1.00 (no increased or reduced risk) for the 95% confidence interval for men, and very nearly (0.97) for women. Thus we are not even at the 95% confidence level for any reduced risk for men, and a value very close to no increased risk appears in the female 95% confidence bound for risk.

Chapter 6: Analysis of variance (ANOVA)

1. The result is significant at $p = 0.0001$, which is highly significant. Thus there would appear to be differences among the three groups.

2. There is a difference between group 2 and both other groups. However, groups 1 and 3 are not significantly different. So European Union countries are different from all the other countries.

3. The significance of any differences disappear when GNP is allowed for, so perhaps the differences are due to GNP, which itself is different (higher) in the European Union.

Chapter 7: Regression

1. WATAGE is below the usual α level of 0.05, but WATBUILD is higher than this value, so we would only accept WATAGE as significant, and therefore a useful predictor.

2. If only using WATAGE, then the formula would be:

WATMOBIL = 0.396 010 × WATAGE + 0.952 785

(the constant 0.952 785 is shown to be significant, and is therefore included).
  using both variables the formula would be:

WATMOBIL = 0.396 010 × WATAGE + 0.133 959 × WATBUILD + 0.952 785

3. $R = 0.121\ 85$, so 12.2% (to one place of decimals).

4. Some method of only keeping significant variables, for example Stepwise.

Chapter 8: Receiver operator characteristic (ROC)

1. The total number of positives (as measured by a gold standard of 1) is 378, and 323 cases are coded 4 or 5. Thus sensitivity = 323/378 or 85% (to the nearest percent).

   The total number of negatives (as measured by a gold standard of 0) is 322, and 77 are coded 4 or 5. Thus specificity = 77/322 or 24% (to the nearest percent).

2. You could add in two arbitrary points where all patients are above a given Waterlow score (zero, for example) so the sensitivity is 1.0 and the false positive rate is also 1.0, and an arbitrarily high score that all patients are below, so both values have to be zero. Then the following graph would be obtained:

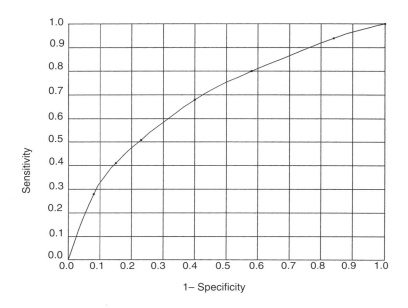

A rough count of the squares (each 0.01 units in area) gives an area of about 0.68 (using squares that are more than half within the line as 0.01, and those less than half within it as 0.0).

Chapter 9: Principal components analysis and factor analysis

1. (a) Three

   (b) Using the rule of ignoring correlations under 0.3, then all variables except DEA20_24 are relevant to the first factor, and only DEA20_24 is relevant to the second factor.

      Using the rule of ignoring those factors that load on more than one factor does not affect the situation, as no factor loads more than 0.3 on both factors.

   (c) Factor 2 is almost purely DEA20_24 and thus this factor relates to the death rate of young men. Factor 1 joins mortality at young age (as measured by INFMORT, NEONATAL and PERINAT) with GDP. I would interpret Factor 1 as representing early death. GDP is shown to be almost a proxy, as the correlations are so high (and negative) for GDP with the factor, and early death is strongly (positively) correlated with it. Factor 2 is young adult male death. The two factors thus model death at different ages.

(d) The only variable loading more than 0.3 is GDP, so this third factor related to money.

Chapter 10: Cluster analysis

1. The Czech Republic seems closer to EU countries, although there are anomalies. For example, Poland is also in this grouping. However, none of the EU countries are in the top seven listed, which are separated from the other countries (mainly EU) by several levels.

2. The formula is (rounded to two significant figures):

$D = (0.0020 \times GDP) + (0.0058 \times INFMORT) - (0.32 \times NEONATAL) +$
$\quad (0.10 \times PERINAT) - 0.50$
$\quad = (0.0020 \times 1500) + (0.0058 \times 17) - (0.32 \times 10) + (0.10 \times 15) - 0.50$
$\quad = 3 + 0.0986 - 3.2 + 1.5 - 0.5$
$\quad = 0.90 \text{ (to two decimal places)}$

Thus Belarus is classified as CEE (incorrectly, as it is part of the former USSR).

Chapter 12: Power analysis

1. The statistical significance is clearly below our conventional α level (0.05), so the result is statistically significant. However, the clinical significance is doubtful, as only 1% ($r^2 = 0.01$) of the variance of one variable is accounted for by the other.

2. Somewhere between 100 and 200 subjects, as the column for effect (0.3) gives $n = 100$ for a power of 0.68 and $n = 200$ for a power of 0.91. As 0.8 is almost in the middle of the range [0.68,0.91], a sample size of about 150 would suffice.

Glossary

α value   The significance at which you say a test result is significant; by convention, this is typically 0.05.

accuracy   A measure of the correctness of the measurement, test, classification, etc., not the same as precision.

adjusted R^2   A conservative measure of the amount of variance accounted for by a regression equation (more conservative than R^2)

agreement   A measure of how much two or more observers give the same result to a mark, classification, etc.

algorithm   A formula or set of rules for computing a result.

Alt   A key on most computer keyboards, used to obtain special functions.

analysis of variance   A test for measuring the significance of the difference in mean values of two or more groups.

ANN   See *artificial neural network*.

ANOVA   Analysis of variance.

artefact   A chance finding that has no real meaning.

artificial neural networks (ANN)   Computer program that attempts to emulate the parallel nature of the human brain.

association   A measure of how much two or more variables are apparently related.

attribute   A measurable item of a larger ensemble of data, e.g. age, height and weight are three attributes of patients.

auto-associative ANN   A self-organizing network, where the input units are also output units

back-propagation   A particular algorithm used in some types of artificial neural network.

Bayesian analysis   A form of analysis employing conditional probabilities. Baye's theorem allows new information to be used to update the conditional probability of an event.

between-group variance   A measure of how different group means are.

binary   Outcomes that take only one of two possible values, e.g. male/female, on/off, yes/no.

bivariate   Relating to two variables.

BMDP   A proprietary statistical software package.

Boltzmann machine   A particular form of artificial neural network used in optimization problems.

Bonferroni inequality   A conservative measure of the probability of occurrence of many pairwise comparisons.

categorical variable   See *nominal variable*.

causality   The concept that one variable influences another in a real sense, as opposed to simply being correlated.

CBL   Computer-based learning (also known as CAL, computer-aided or computer assisted learning).

centroid clustering   A clustering algorithm.

chi square (χ^2)   A test of independence of nominal variables.

click   Depression of the mouse key.

clinical significance   A measure of how much a result actually matters in clinical practice. This is not necessarily the same as statistical significance.

cluster analysis   A set of techniques for categorizing data into clusters that are hopefully meaningfully related.

coefficient   A number used to quantify the amount of some variable.

coefficient of determination   The square of the correlation coefficient (r^2). It gives the amount of variance accounted for by the correlation coefficient.

Cohen's kappa (κ)   A measure of agreement between two observers.

communality   In factor analysis, the variance of the variables accounted for by the factors identified.

concurrent validity   Where groups are known to differ with respect to some construct, then a measure of that construct is said to show concurrent validity if that measure identifies a difference.

conditional probability   The probability of event B occurring given that event A has occurred.

confidence levels or limits   A range of values within which you have a given level of confidence of a given parameter, e.g. a 95% confidence interval for a mean value is the range of values within which you are 95% sure the real mean lies.

constant   A value that does not vary.

construct validity   The ability to measure some trait, e.g. intelligence.

content validity   A measure of the relevance of an item.

contingency table   A table showing the frequencies of all possible values of a variable or several variables.

convergence   In artificial neural networks and other optimization techniques, where the successive iterations show little change in the solution.

convergent validity   The means whereby the measure is tested for harmonization with some preexisting measure.

correlation   The degree to which two variables are linearly related.

correspondence analysis   An advanced method of showing relationships among categorical (nominal) variables.

covariate   In ANOVA, a variable that is accounted for in an analysis of two or more other variables.

Cramer's V   A correlation coefficient used in nominal variables.

criterion-related validity   How well a new instrument compares to some well tried older measure.

Cronbach alpha (α)   A measure of internal reliability.

dataset   A collection of data, usually of several variables.

decubitus ulcer   A sore caused by pressure damage.

degrees of freedom   A measure of the quantity of data, used to calibrate the test result for significance.

dendrograms   A graphical display of cluster analysis; an alternative to icicle plots.

denominator   The bottom part of a fraction.

density search techniques   A form of cluster analysis.

dependent variable   A variable the value of which is assumed to be the result of some other variable(s).

dialogue box   Computer display where the user is requested to enter data or make a decision.

dimensions   A measure of the number of meaningful variables in a dataset.

directory   A named place in the computer's store where files may be placed.

discriminant analysis   A linear method of allocating members to a group.

discriminant equation   The equation in discriminant analysis that defines group membership.

divergent validity   A measure of how different concepts discriminate.

double click   Two rapid depressions of the mouse button.

effect   A measure of the practical (clinical significance) outcome of a test, as opposed to statistical significance.

eigenvectors   A variable of an orthogonal set of variables (i.e. variables that are not correlated with each other) that describe a dataset.

equivalence   The concept that describes measures of agreement between two observers.

Euclidean space   Three-dimensional space.

expected values   In contingency tables, the frequencies you would expect if the variables were independent of each other.

external reliability   Measures of stability or equivalence.

extrapolation   Using a formula beyound the range in which it is known to be appropriate.

F **ratio**   A test statistic used in ANOVA.

face validity   A priori relevance of an item.

factor analysis   An analysis that tries to ascertain the number of dimensions of a dataset using linear methods.

factors   The dimensions resulting from a factor analysis.

false-negative rate   The ratio of classifications wrongly ascribed negative to all truly positive classifications.

false-positive rate   The ratio of classifications wrongly ascribed positive to all truly negative classifications.

files   In computing, data stored under one name in a directory.

Fisher's exact test   A more robust, but computationally expensive, alternative to the χ^2 test.

fitness   In genetic algorithms, the performance of a (synthetic) gene on a given task.

flooding   In artificial neural networks, when a unit gets stuck at a value due to excessive inputs from other units.

Friedman's test   A non-parametric equivalent to repeated-measures ANOVA.

function key   A specialized key on the computer keyboard that performs some task.

Generalizability   In artificial neural networks, the ability of a solution to work on new data.

GENESIS   A genetic algorithm software package (there is also a neural network package of the same name).

genetic algorithm   An optimization technique using concepts borrowed form evolutionary biology.

gold standard   In receiver operating characteristic, the classification that is believed to be true.

gradient   In graphs, the slope of a line.

harmonic mean   Used in power analysis to allow groups of different sizes to be evaluated.

hetero-associative ANNs   Neural networks that have distinct inputs and outputs.

heteroscedasticity   The opposite of homoscedasticity.

hidden layers   Units in artificial neural networks that receive no direct input, and give no direct output.

histogram   A bar chart that shows the frequencies of ranges of some (at least ordinal) variable.

homoscedasticity   Where the points about a regression show no pattern, in the sense that the range of data is the same at each point on the line.

Hopfield nets   A particular form of auto-associative neural network.

hypertext   A form of electronic document that contains cross-references to other electronic documents, which may be accessed directly, typically by means of the mouse key.

hypothesis   A statement that is capable of being tested using quantitative methods.

icicle plot   A graphical display of cluster analysis; an alternative to a dendrogram.

icon   A graphical depiction of some utility on the computer screen.

independence   A measure of how variables are not correlated or related to each other.

independent variable   The variable that is assumed to be the cause rather than effect of some other variable(s).

inferential statistical tests   Those that test some hypothesis.

initial parameters   In optimization techniques (e.g. neural networks) the values of the start-up variables.

instrument   A device used to collect data, e.g. questionnaire, interview schedule, laboratory equipment.

internal reliability   A measure of the extent to which several items measure the same thing (e.g. in a questionnaire).

interquartile range   The 50% of values in the centre of a distribution, from the 25th percentile to the 75th percentile.

inter-rater reliability   The extent to which two observers agree.

intervening variables   Where one variable effects a second variable, which itself effects a third variable.

intra-class correlation coefficient   The correlation coefficient when employed to give a value of repeatability.

Kaiser's criterion   A criterion for retaining principal components, i.e. where eigenvalues are over 1.0.

kappa (κ)   See *Cohen's kappa (κ)*.

Kendal's tau (τ)   An alternative to Spearman rank correlation coefficient for correlation testing of non-normal data.

K-means clustering   A method of cluster analysis; particularly useful for very large data sets.

Kohonen net   A form of self-organizing neural network.

Kolmogorov–Smirnov goodness of fit test   A test of distributions, typically used to test for normality.

Kruskal–Wallis test   A non-parametric equivalent to ANOVA.

learning rate   A parameter used in neural networks.

Levene's test for equality of variances   A prior test used in independent Student's *t*-test SPSS to determine if the variances of the two groups are different.

linearity   Any relation able to be modelled as a straight line in a graph of one variable against the other.

local minima   A suboptimal solution for an optimization technique.

logistic regression   A regression technique for use on a binary dependent variable.

Macintosh   A type of microcomputer.

mainframe   A multi-user computer.

Mann–Whitney test   A non-parametric equivalent to Student's *t*-test for independent groups.

matrix   A table of coefficients of one or more variables.

McNemar's test   A test for differences of paired nominal data.

mean   The 'average' value obtained by summing all values and dividing by the number of values.

median   The 'average' value obtained by selecting the middle value in an ordered list.

median clustering   A form of cluster analysis.

menu   A list of options from which the user of a computer package selects.

metric   A measure of distance.

microcomputer   A personal computer.

Microsoft Windows (trademark Microsoft)   A graphical interface used in IBM-compatible microcomputers.

Minitab   A proprietary statistical software package.

mode   The 'average' value obtained by selecting the most common value. There may be more than one mode for any given distribution.

moderated relationships   Where a relationship holds for some categories of a variable, but not all.

momentum   An initial parameter for neural networks that increases stability.

mouse   A device on a computer for accessing graphical interfaces.

MS-DOS (trademark Microsoft)   An operating system used on IBM-compatible PCs.

multilayer perceptron   A perceptron with at least one hidden layer.

multiple analysis of variance (MANOVA)   An extension of ANOVA to more than one dependent variable.

multiple causation   Where for an effect there is more than one cause.

multiple pairwise comparisons   Where several tests are made between pairs of groups.

multiple regression   An extension of regression for more than one independent variable.

noise   Data from random events that are nothing to do with the effect being measured.

nominal variable   Also called categorical variable. A variable that can only take non-overlapping values that have no intrinsic numerical meaning and can only be used to identify a category (e.g. male/female).

nominator   Top part of a fraction.

non-linear   Not able to be modelled as linear.

non-parametric   To do with distributions that are not normal.

non-parametric tests   Tests that do not assume normal distributions.

normalized   Data constrained to lie in a given range (typically [0,1] or [−1, +1]).

normally distributed   A distribution the frequency histogram of which shows a characteristic bell-shaped curve.

NP-complete problem   An NP-complete problem is one that has three main features. It is simple to define the problem, it is easy to solve the problem when the problem is small, but it very quickly becomes impossible to solve, even in principle, as the problem grows in size.

null hypothesis   An hypothesis stated in such a form that no differences or no correlation, etc., are expected.

oblique rotation   A particular manipulation of the factors in factor analysis to allow easier interpretation.

odds ratio   The relative risk of the occurrence of some (typically nominal) outcome given the value of some other (typically nominal) variable.

one-tailed test   A test where you are only interested in results in one direction, e.g. a positive correlation rather than a positive or negative one.

one-way ANOVA   ANOVA where only one independent variable is used.

optimization technique   Iterative technique for producing a solution that may not be (and usually is not) optimal.

ordinal data   Continuous data where successive intervals do not necessarily have the same interpretation. For example, in a race the difference between first and second place is not, in general, the same as that between second and third places.

outlier   A data point that is a long way from the main part of the distribution.

overfitting/overtraining   Where a solution goes past a generalizable solution to fit the training test data better but the test data worse.

p **value**   The probability of a test result occurring by chance.

parameter   In distributions, a value that describes the distribution.

parametric   Pertaining to normal distributions.

partial correlation   Correlation between two variables, after allowing for one or more additional variables.

pattern   Set of data used to input to a neural network.

pattern matching   A technique of identifying complex data.

Pearson's correlation coefficient   A parametric correlation test.

perceptron   A particular design of a hetero-associative neural network.

phi (ϕ) test   A correlation test for 2×2 contingency tables.

population   All the possible subjects from which a sample may be drawn.

population variance   A measure of the dispersion in a population.

post hoc tests   Tests performed after the main test, in particular to test differences between the group means in ANOVA.

power   The ability of a test to reject the null hypothesis correctly.

power curves   Graphical displays of the power of tests.

precision   A measure of repeatability.

predictive validity   Where a test is applied and the group followed up to determine whether the test can predict those subjects who will develop some condition.

principal components   The dimensions of a dataset that account for the largest amount of variance.

principal components analysis   A particular form of factor analysis.

prior probability   The probability of an event occurring in a population when no particular extra knowledge is given.

pulmonary embolism   When a blood clot (thrombosis) becomes mobile (embolus) and lodges in the lung circulation.

quadratic   A relationship that is based on squared data.

qualitative   Data that cannot be placed into closed lists prior to analysis.

random selection   Where each member of a population has an equal chance of being selected in a sample.

ratio data   Continuous data where, in addition to being interval data, there is a concept of absolute zero, and ratios are meaningful (e.g. a blood sugar level of 6.0 is twice a blood sugar level of 3.0).

receiver operating characteristic   A technique for measuring sensitivity and specificity at different thresholds.

relative risk   See *odds ratio*.

reliability   To do with the repeatability of a test.

repeated-measures ANOVA   ANOVA for matched data.

research question   A concise statement of what the research is attempting to find out.

Return key   Key used to enter data or produce carriage returns on the keyboard.

rotation   One of many possible manipulations of factors to make them easier to comprehend.

sample   A (usually random) selection from a population.

sample variance   A measure of the variability of the sample.

SAS   A proprietary statistical software package.

scatterplot   A graph where one variable is plotted against another; the x and y values of each item are plotted as points.

scintigrams   A medical image created using radioisotopes.

scroll bar   A device on the edge of a window allowing you to move up or down and left or and right within the window.

sensitivity   The ratio of true-positive results to all positive results; synonymous with true-positive rate.

Sheffé's test   A post hoc test for determining which, if any, of pairs of groups have significantly different means.

sign test   A non-parametric test that determines if two (paired) measurements are significantly different from each other.

significance   See *statistical significance* and *clinical significance*.

simple Euclidean distance   The distance between two points in three-dimensional space.

simulated annealing   A particular form of optimization based on the mathematics of crystal freezing.

Spearman rank test   A non-parametric equivalent to Pearson's correlation test.

specificity   The ratio of true-negative results to all negative results; synonymous with true-negative rate.

split-half test   A test of internal reliability.

SPSS   A proprietary statistics package (the assumed package for this book).

spurious correlations   Where two variables show a correlation, but are themselves related.

stability   Where a test is able to give a similar result repeatedly.

standard deviation   A measure of variability useful in normal distributions.

standard error of the mean (SEM)   A measure of the variability of the means of samples.

statistical significance   A measure of the probability of obtaining a given test result by chance alone; not necessarily the same a clinical significance.

Statview   A proprietary statistical software package.

STEPS   A suite of statistical CBL packages from The Teaching and Learning Technology Programme.

stepwise regression   A regression method whereby only significant variables are kept in the regression equation.

structure matrix   A matrix consisting of the correlations of each of the variables with the factors derived in a factor analysis.

Student's *t*-test   A special case of ANOVA for two groups.

synthetic genes   A mathematical entity used in genetic algorithms to emulate the behaviour of genes.

Teaching and Learning Technology Programme (TLTP)   A (UK) Government backed initiative to produce high-quality educational CBL packages for higher education.

transformation   Mathematical formula used typically to make analysis easier by changing a non-linear or non-normal variable to a linear or normal variable.

travelling salesman problem   An NP-complete problem, the shortest path linking many cities.

true-negative rate   Ratio of number of subjects correctly identified as not having a condition to the total number of subjects not having the condition.

true-positive rate   Ratio of the number of subjects correctly identified as having a condition to the total number of subjects having the condition.

two-tailed test   A test where you are only interested in results in either direction, e.g. a positive correlation or a positive or negative one.

two-way ANOVA   ANOVA using two independent variables.

type I error   Where a test reports a significant result that in fact occurred by chance, i.e. the null hypothesis is rejected but is in fact true.

type II error   Where a test reports a result as occurring by chance that in fact it did not, i.e. the null hypothesis is accepted but is in fact false.

unexplained variance   The residual variance not accounted for by the analysis.

unsupervised learning   Where neural networks organize themselves without training.

validity   The concept of the appropriateness of a technique to solve the problem.

variables   Items that can be measured and help describe an individual in a sample.

variance   The square of the standard deviation.

varimax   A method used to simplify the interpretation of factors in factor analysis.

Waterlow score   A risk assessment score for decubitus ulcers.

weights   In neural networks, the strength of linkage between units.

Wilcoxon test   A non-parametric equivalent to Student's paired t-test.

window   A rectangular portion of the screen in which a computer program may run.

Windows '95   (trademark Microsoft) A replacement for Windows that does not need MS-DOS to run.

Windows 3.11   (trademark Microsoft) The last version of windows to run under MS-DOS.

Word for Windows   (trademark Microsoft)   A word processing software package.

Yate's correction   A refinement to the χ^2 test.

Index

DATE DUE